The Power of DRES

DRES System's Guide to Building a Professional Image and Working Wardrobe

Margaret Spencer, DRES System Founder
with Brenda Azevedo
Colleen Bradley
Kira Brown
Lori Goddard-Weed
Cheryl Michaels
Melissa Sabatine
Kat Smith
and Corey Urbina

The material in this book is intended for educational purposes only. No expressed implied guarantee as to the effects of the use of the recommendations can be given nor liability taken. This book does not guarantee any results.

ISBN: 978-0-9859547-1-0
Library of Congress Control Number: 2012914437

Printed in the United States of America
Cover Photo by Tara Gimmer at La Ree Boutique in Bellevue, Washington

www.DRESsystem.com

holobi.

We bought this for your Christmas because we so proud and wanted you each to have your own personalized copy from Colleen.

Love MOM & DAD

December 2012

To all those who seek image confidence
and aspire to reach their full potential

CONTENTS

INTRODUCTION

By Margaret Spencer

Everyone deserves to feel attractive and confident. It's a fundamental need to want others to like and accept us. The challenge in feeling confident is that there is often a large gap between who we want to be and where we are currently.

Together, some of my most talented stylists and I decided to write our book to bridge this gap and share with you insights into the DRES System: How you can tap into your power, and why we feel the DRES System is the most powerful form of styling to bring out your inner and outer beauty. You will get an inside look at working with our DRES System–Certified Stylists, pick up some styling tips and, hopefully, relate to some of our quirky stories. You will see that we all share wardrobe challenges, body insecurities, and the quest for confidence.

For me in particular, it has been a long road to possessing a confident and pulled-together image. When I was growing up, I remember being eleven years old and idolizing Farrah Fawcett. I would watch the TV program *Charlie's Angels* and be in awe of these beautiful women who were smart (so-called detectives), powerful (packing iron), and beautiful (thought they woke up looking like that). I loved everything about Farrah: her glamorous wardrobe; her long, lanky and tan figure; her broad smile and, most of all, her perfect hair. So I ripped a photo out of a magazine and asked my mom to take me to my very first professional hairstyling appointment in a salon where I, in all honesty, believed this woman would magically transform me into Farrah with one haircut. When she was done, I was thrilled by the transformation from all-one-length, little-girl hair to the new and sophisticated look the stylist gave me.

The first time I tried to style this cut on my own, it dawned on me that this was not going to be easy. I needed to buy a curling iron and learn how to use it. My first attempts looked like two horns coming out of my temples, much more like a musk ox than Farrah's elegant, soft curls. My mother had a large family portrait made that year that hung in our living room, so I had a hard time forgetting about this awkward phase for years to come. What I lacked was styling techniques.

A few years later, I finally mastered the feathered-hair look with the help of a permanent wave and lots of practice. It was now the early 1980s, and there was a new fashion trend that I just had to have: a pair of baggies. This is a pant cut that is the opposite of my body shape. Baggies have a narrow waist, full hips, and tapered legs. Add to that pleats in front that add bulk! Full of excitement for this new trend, I couldn't wait to go to Nordstrom to try on this new look. With my thick waist, full tummy, and straight hips, in the dressing room it quickly became clear that this pant did not work for my figure. It seemed this pant was designed for Barbie. Not being a person who gives up quickly when it come to things I really want, I assessed my options: I could buy the smaller size that fit in the hips and not button the waist or buy the larger size that buttoned but made me look like a clown. Because I got great joy in being the first to wear what I knew would be a big trend, I just had to have them. So I chose the baggies that I could barely button at the waist. I wore them all school year, even though they gave me stomachaches. I'm sharing this story with you so that you'll know what it feels like to be a true fashion victim who chases every trend. I realize now that you should always dress to bring out your personal best and not mindlessly follow trends. You will always look the most chic and attractive in items that complement you.

Flash forward to 2006. I'm now a devoted mom, with two beautiful daughters, who is dedicated to teaching my girls to be smart, powerful, and beautiful. As I look back, this is much like my impression of the characters from *Charlie's Angels*. I have gone to great efforts to teach both of them to have a great self-image, to enrich their lives in every way, and to show them how knowledge is power. This appeared to be working wonderfully as they excelled in school and were fearless when acting in school stage productions or speaking in class.

As they were becoming teenagers, I began to see a decline. Not only did I witness a big drop in their self-confidence, but they also started to look at themselves more critically. Like any good mom, I wanted both of my daughters to have a good self-image and body image. Now that they were growing into teens, suddenly insecurities emerged. They were comparing their bodies to other girls' and to one another. I asked my daughters to share their thoughts with you on how they feel about their body shapes. With this example of opposing body challenges, I hope this helps you realize that no matter what shape you have, we all struggle with some amount of insecurities about our shape.

Body Image: From the Perspective of "the Skinny Girl"

My older daughter was born with a very thin build—and not just narrow. All of her bones are long and slender in shape, too. Her metabolism is such that she can eat anything and never gain weight. You may think that this is ideal and she should have a great body image. Not the case. Her body image issues are centered around being so thin that she lacks curves, which she sees on most of the other girls at school, and that her little sister has. She struggles to find clothes that will fit her figure and are not cut for curvier girls.

Now eighteen, she says, "There is a misconception among women that if you're built to be skinny you have hit the jackpot of appearance. Although skinny is presented as what every girl should want to attain, actually being skinny does not guarantee self-confidence or promise a lack of body issues because even skinny girls don't look like Barbie. As a girl built to be skinny, it has been difficult for me to feel womanly or sexy. What comes with skinny isn't guaranteed beauty but rather a small chest, sticklike limbs and a tendency to look like either a guy or a little kid. I don't have the curves that, according to the Dove® Campaign, make you a 'real woman,' and I look more like the skinny models being called unnatural and sickly. I just want to be thought of as healthy and normal. But I've had to accept that this is who I am: that just because I'm thin doesn't mean I have an eating disorder, that not having curves doesn't make me less of a woman."

Body Image: From the Perspective of "the Athletic Girl"

My younger daughter has a very different body shape from her sister. She has a larger bone structure, not as much in height as in width. While she is not overweight, she simply has larger, broader bones and a small waist. Add to that lots of muscles, as she is a very competitive soccer player. In addition, as she grew into a teenager, she developed more womanly curves. Her clothing challenges are finding clothes that fit over her athletic/curvy shape and don't make her appear larger than she really is.

Now at fifteen she says, "Being an elite athlete I have always been bigger than other girls. I've watched my more dainty friends drop the sport because they got knocked around too much; because of this I have always been grateful that I have such a strong, athletic build. My bones are big, I'm decently tall, and I'm pretty much stronger than all of my girlfriends, and a lot of my guy friends. My body type makes me a tough player; however, starting in junior high school I started to become self-conscious of the way I looked. Other girls I know are small, and graceful. No matter if they're curvy or not, they generally have a delicate look. I'm not petite, and I never will be, and I guess that is why it's difficult for me to think of myself as beautiful because all the girls everyone says are pretty are always small. Everywhere you look what is considered pretty is a 'slender' model.

"I do not have voluptuous curves, and I'm not chubby, I'm just burly, and there is no one telling me that that is beautiful. I think why it's hard for me to understand how I feel about myself is because I don't want to be 'smaller' like a model, or less muscular. My body type has helped me become the athlete I want to be, but I still want to feel pretty.

"Sometimes my friends complain about their weight, which really everyone does. So when they do this, I joke about how I weigh so much more, and they just say 'I don't count,' and it's all lighthearted, and it makes sense, but it just shows how there isn't really any consideration of what strong girls are supposed to be like."

In my effort to help my daughters embrace their shapes and value their uniqueness, I became more aware of the confusing messages our society sends to women. Distorted body shapes are still parading the runway, and fashion magazines display digitally enhanced bodies that are unobtainable by most. It's pretty tough to accept yourself and embrace your body shape when you're told you are a triangle or pear. This heightened my awareness of the need for positive, healthy body images that women could relate to which help us accept the body shapes we are born with.

Today, our culture has started to embrace diversity more, yet we are still lacking positive methods to help us describe and accept our diverse body shapes. This is why I committed myself to creating positive image associations for not only my daughters but for all women. My first thought was that women need the right tools and support to help them feel confident and accept themselves the way they are made. It's important for me that my daughters and all women learn that their bodies are not wrong—it's the clothes that are wrong for them. So the first place I started was with the labels we use to identify our body shapes. Because I want all women to value themselves, I came up with the gem analogy for body shapes. The concept that everybody is a precious gem became the foundation of my company.

Over the last six years I have refined this system and taught it to several other women who wanted to become independent personal stylists so that they too could share this concept with their clients. Our national team of specially trained, certified DRES Stylists provides you with the support you desire. They are not here to just polish your image—they also share my belief that inner confidence is part of styling. Our stylists will show you your beauty in a brand-new way and help you to build the wardrobe of your dreams.

With this book in hand, we wish you more personal power. We welcome you to the world of the DRES System. It is my wholehearted hope that you feel more confident and empowered after reading this book.

CHAPTER 1

DRES SYSTEM

Where Fashion, Art, and Science Mingle

By Margaret Spencer

That dreaded question. It races through your mind every morning as you stand there half-awake staring at a closetful of clothes. It's the first decision of the day, and it can set the tone for the next twenty-four hours. What to wear?

> *"What you wear is how you present yourself to the world, especially today, when human contacts are so quick. Fashion is instant language."*
> —Miuccia Prada

With a well-laid-out wardrobe plan, deciding what to wear can be a breeze. All you need to do is choose an outfit that is appropriate for your day's activities. Your image is nonverbal communication. Just like a billboard, you have only seconds to communicate who you are when you meet someone for the first time or greet someone in passing. The first time we see someone we make judgments about them, regardless of how hard we try to avoid stereotyping other people. We look at their eyes and face; then scan their overall appearance and land at their shoes before circling back up. We evaluate them on our own very subjective scale of attractiveness, and decide if they will be friendly. We size up character and professionalism. Know that your nonverbal image speaks volumes—so make sure yours says professional, credible, trustworthy, and likable.

Most importantly, your verbal and nonverbal messages about yourself should be consistent. Your verbal message is how you present yourself with words; your nonverbal message is your appearance. If your words are saying, "I'm a CEO," and your image is saying "librarian," there can be a disconnect for people. Your appearance is your most powerful nonverbal communication tool, so you can't afford not to get it right. If your verbal and nonverbal messages do not align, you can come off as unprofessional or, even worse, dishonest. Just as Miuccia Prada suggests, fashion is language. Reading this book will show you how to master the language of fashion so that you can reach your full potential.

YOUR FULL POTENTIAL

When you were born, not only were you born perfect, you also possessed immense potential. Your potential represents your ability to achieve what you want out of life. I wish for you to become your best self and ultimately reach your full potential by mastering your image. Too often I see women who possess so much potential that they are not harnessing. So many great features not played up, great figures hidden in the wrong clothes, beautiful natural coloring dulled by poor color choices—all of these things steal your brilliance.

Potential for greatness lies within all of us. How we feel about ourselves carries over into all other areas of our lives. Not only in the visual sense but also for all other areas of our lives: for example, the way people respond to each other and, most importantly, the way they feel about and treat each other.

As I write this, my younger daughter is finishing up her last year in junior high school. I don't know about you, but being around teens always makes me reflect on my own teenage experience. I remember the first day of school in ninth grade. I was feeling very confident now that I was an upperclassman, and the fact that I had a new back-to-school outfit on didn't hurt, either. I was sitting in drama class waiting for the teacher to arrive and, after thirty minutes, we realized the teacher might never come. Instead of notifying the office staff, we all just got busy socializing in the auditorium. It was drama class, after all.

Not having friends in the class, I grew bored and noticed a shy-looking girl sitting by herself a few seats away. I thought to myself, "Why would she wear clothes that look like her mom bought from a discount store and not even try to style her hair? Why?"

In the middle of my teen years, when image was so important to me, I struggled with understanding why she did not put in any effort. Underneath it all, I could tell that she had lots of potential. She had a rather slender build, considered attractive by most, a nicely balanced figure, and a face with good bone structure. In case you're wondering, yes, I did notice these types of details, even at this age.

Remembering that I had my full cosmetic bag in my dark purple LeSportsac purse (you '80s girls will remember this *it* bag made of parachute material). I thought to myself *surely she would like to look "totally glam."* She just didn't know how. So I asked her if I could do her makeup. She sheepishly said "sure," quickly realizing she had nothing else to do and nothing to lose.

After her hair-and-makeup mini-makeover, the popular kids in the class came circling around and complimented her on how great she looked. Later that day I saw her walking down the halls and receiving even more compliments and attention. There was something distinctly different in her walk and she seemed to glow from the inside.

I was glowing, too. I remember feeling so powerful that I could cause this chain reaction in her confidence and, in turn, the way others treated her. The teacher never did show up that day, but I still learned an important lesson: empowering others empowers you.

Sometimes a transformation stems from changes on the outside, and it can forever change that person, inside. Other times, it's the other way around, and the person changes on the inside so that the outside appearance has to catch up with the new, inner persona. It doesn't matter in which direction it happens—it's an empowering experience. There is nothing like the feeling of making a personal breakthrough in life.

Following is my favorite quote about reaching your full potential, which I hope will inspire you as much as it does me. Whether or not you are spiritual, I hope you can receive this powerful message.

> *Our deepest fear is not that we are inadequate. Our deepest fear is that we are powerful beyond measure. It is our light, not our darkness, that most frightens us. We ask ourselves, who am I to be brilliant, gorgeous, talented, and fabulous? Actually, who are you not to be? You are a child of God. Your playing small doesn't serve the world. There's nothing enlightened about shrinking so that other people won't feel insecure around you. We are all meant to shine, as children do. We are born to make manifest the glory of God that is within us. It's not just in some of us, it's in everyone. And as we let our own light shine, we unconsciously give other people permission to do the same. As we are liberated from our own fear, our presence automatically liberates others.*
>
> —Marianne Williamson

So let your light shine by owning your beauty both inside and out. Step into the power of your image, and honor your full potential!

WHO IS BEAUTIFUL?

You are beautiful! All people possess beauty. The human body in and of itself is a thing of marvel and beauty. When you were born, you came into this world as a perfect little bundle of joy that mesmerized your parents. Now you have the potential to attract a new kind of attention.

The way I see it, people are like gemstones found naturally in the earth. Have you ever seen one? It looks like a rough rock on the outside, almost like a lump of coal to discard. When it's cracked open, you see its brilliance in rough form. Then the gem is polished and displayed in just the right way: with facets that pick up the light, sparkling and showing off its best assets. Any flaws are rarely noticed. They are pale in comparison to this shiny object perched atop a shiny gold setting. We're all diamonds in the rough. Polish your image to reveal your brilliance.

Just like a precious gemstone, each woman is unique with her own personal qualities. In gemstones this is referred to as the four *c*'s: cut, color, clarity, and carat. In the DRES Personal Styling System, this translates into body shape, skin tone, fashion style, and clothing size. This makes up your Personal DRES Profile. Once we have a better understanding of you, we can help you look and feel radiant.

Gemstones and the DRES Profile

Cut = **Body Shape**

Color = **Skin Tone**

Clarity = **Fashion Style**

Carat = **Clothing Size**

It's easy to look at a person with a shape different than ours and think *they have it so much better*. The truth is that each shape has characteristics that are meant to be highlighted and others that are better to conceal. The goal is to embrace our shape and the gifts it brings, while balancing our figure.

Look for current styles that fit your own Personal DRES System Profile. After all, when others view us, they look for the balance and harmony in your overall appearance. As with precious stones, we have a few perceived imperfections; however, when we highlight our assets, our brilliance outshines them.

"We spend far too much time and energy contemplating our inadequacies. We forget that we are all perfect in our imperfection."

—Kate Dillon, plus-size model

DRES SYSTEM PROFILE

"It all starts in the morning, having clothing options that match your mood and the weather, knowing with confidence that your choices complement your look and body. My wife gets ready for work in half the time and has a positive and energetic attitude as she starts her day. That positive attitude and energy is transferred to those around her and all benefit."

—Andrew Walter, a client's husband

When you embrace your unique beauty and recognize your full potential, you can attract the right people and opportunities by creating the right image. Use the power in your appearance as leverage to meet the right people and further your career.

In business the old saying "dress for success" is not just a cliché. This was first seen as the title of a 1975 book by John T. Molloy about the effect of clothing on a person's success in their business and personal life. My belief is that you should always dress like your company's management if you want to make it to the top. When people see you dressed professionally, they hold more respect for you. They see that you have a lot of respect for yourself and take care and pride in your appearance. This sends a powerful message that you are on your way to the top.

Getting dressed for work does not mean having to lose your personal style. As long as you understand how to achieve a polished and professional look, you will be on the path of living up to your full potential. Your main objective in getting dressed for work is to project a competent image. Anything that would be better suited for the beach or a nightclub would not send the message that you are serious about your chosen profession. Appropriate clothing is a sign that people can trust you to make good choices. Any clothing or accessories that are too casual will erode others' confidence in you. And if your style choices are too loud in color or pattern, they are distractions to doing business. You wouldn't wear Jimmy Choo heels while rock climbing or a Donna Karan gown golfing, so why wear

Lululemon Athletica yoga wear or a fluorescent yellow, American Apparel T-shirt to work?

In relationships this also speaks for you. When you're wearing your ultimate colors and your clothing looks tailor-made, you come off as someone who has it all together, someone people want to know. People tend to gravitate toward and want to associate with those who are going places. Whether you are attracting friends or partners, knowing the tricks of styling will open up opportunities.

Color plays a big part in attracting important people to you. If you wear a color that looks poorly on you, people pick up on this. They may not readily recognize why they feel put off or understand what it is that bothers them. It may be a feeling that something isn't authentic. They may think that you are not feeling well or that you're just plain dull.

When your colors are aligned, people are attracted to you. There is a glow about you. Not only are they drawn to your harmony and balance, they also notice your brilliance. The right colors not only enhance your appearance—they support your image and bring out the best in you.

PERCEIVED INTELLIGENCE

There is a shared perception in our culture that attractive people are more intelligent and competent. When you look put together on the outside, you appear to have it all put together on the inside, too. Your ability to make good choices on your appropriate style, color, and fit reflects your perceived decision-making ability. I'd like to make it clear that physical attractiveness is not a "born with it or not" kind of thing but, rather, how you learn and decide to present yourself.

There was an interesting study mentioned in a *Psychology Today* article from March 29, 2009, by Satoshi Kanazawa, Ph.D. He uses evolutionary psychology to analyze social sciences. He notes that "people believe beautiful people are more intelligent, because they in fact are."

In this article he mentions that the National Longitudinal Study of Adolescent Health, conducted by a team of researchers at the University of North Carolina–Chapel Hill, is one of the very few social science data sets that take seriously the biological and genetic influences on human behavior. As a result, they routinely measure both the intelligence and physical attractiveness of their test subjects. Their test results showed a clear association between the degree of physical attractiveness with their test subjects' intelligence.

In another *Psychology Today* article from 2010, Satoshi Kanazawa takes this a little further by saying, "Everybody knows that intelligence and education are very highly correlated. What they don't know is that physical attractiveness is equally highly correlated with intelligence as education is. If you want to estimate someone's intelligence without giving them an IQ test, you would do just as well to base your estimate on their physical attractiveness as you would to base it on their years of education."

With this new understanding of the correlation between intellect and image, I feel that individualized style education should be taught in all educational institutions.

Unfortunately, this is not currently the case. This is why I have taken a subject that has been surrounded by mystery and sifted it down into an easy-to-understand program that empowers each individual with the tools and support they need to discover how to reach their full potential of attractiveness.

All women can achieve perceived beauty and intelligence through skilled styling. It's really all about learning what works for you, and then developing an authentic look that is in balance with who you are on the inside and out. Anyone can be perceived as beautiful through educated style choices. Just look at Marilyn Monroe. She was just Norma Jean until she underwent a complete makeover. There was extensive planning and strategy to create her new look. Everything about her was styled: her name was changed, her hair was dyed platinum blonde, her lips were painted red, her eyes were lined with upturned eyeliner tips and adorned with two half-strips of false lashes. Her wardrobe was carefully selected. And don't forget the famous beauty mark above her lip. Yes, this, too, was penciled in. Both Marilyn Monroe and her team of stylists perfected her image throughout her short career. Fifty years later, she is still considered the most iconic symbol of American beauty.

Just like Marilyn, you are your brand. From my years working in corporate communications and corporate branding for large companies such as Nike® and Intel®, I realized that personal image is also no different than a company's brand. Developing any kind of brand involves research, analysis, and goal setting. While working on corporate branding, my design team and I spent a lot of time and care crafting a thick corporate style-guide manual that would ensure brand consistency so that our corporate image and message would come across the way it was intended. Inside these style guides were measurements, specifications, instructions on proper color usage, and myriad other dos and don'ts.

Each of us can develop our own personal brand with a detailed style guide of what works and what doesn't for our individual features and proportions. There is no way that one item will look good on everyone because we are all so unique in our shape and coloring. Beware of those who say, "This looks good on everyone." Few items truly do.

Because of how our appearance plays an enormous role in our lives, like getting a good job, meeting a partner/spouse, to even getting better service in a restaurant, you should have a solid understanding of how the nonverbal messages you choose are translated to others. I want to help you understand what brings out the best in you and make it easy to find clothing that matches your objective.

It's important to think about how we want to present ourselves to the world each day. Your words, your actions, and your visual presentation all need to come together and be consistent for people to build trust in you. Getting clear on your personal brand, and then presenting a balanced and confident image is the key to attracting the people and success you desire.

BALANCE AND CONFIDENCE

"I wanted to let you know that I absolutely LOVE my clothes and have gotten wonderful comments on everything that I have been wearing. It is amazing the confidence I have when wearing something I love and I know looks good on me. I have not only gotten comments on how good the clothes look, but how good I look, and some people have even noticed a different confidence about me by the way I am carrying myself when wearing them. I am actually looking forward to going shopping again."

—Kristi Walter, Client EC9 (Emerald, Chic, Color Code 9)

I believe that beauty is found in balance and confidence. These are the fundamental principles on which the DRES System educational program is based.

Balance in the alignment of your outer image with your inner image is one part of balance. The other part is to achieve visual balance in your silhouette's proportions. We use visual illusion techniques with color, line, and form to bring your image into balance. There are hundreds of scientific studies indicating that the human brain is programmed to respond positively to balance and symmetry.

Confidence is key because this sends a message to others that you believe you are beautiful and worthy. You have to see yourself this way first before others will follow suit. A beautiful person on the outside without inner confidence is simply a pretty facade. When you let your true authentic self shine through and you believe you look your best, your brilliance is unmatched. Ask yourself if you possess these qualities:

Balance

- Visual balance in your image
- Both inner and outer beauty
- Balance in all areas of your life

Confidence

- Projecting an image you intend
- An image authentic to you
- Self-esteem and self-acceptance

Everyone possesses their own unique beauty and authentic style. It's our job as DRES System Personal Stylists to bring out that beauty for the world to see by helping you obtain more balance and confidence. As trained personal stylists, we teach that confidence in who we are comes from self-acceptance. A balanced image and a balanced life go a long way toward building this confidence.

"But the most important lesson is to bring beauty to your attitude."
—Dixie Carter, actress

GOLDEN RATIO

Enhanced beauty is achieved through science and mathematics. What? Yes, things we consider to be beautiful can be explained by the science of balance and proportions. The golden ratio is a math-based formula for visual balance that has been discovered to appear in nature and in the human body. It suggests that things with a ratio of 1:1.618 tend to be the most pleasing to the eye. An example of the golden ratio in nature is the distance between each curve on a seashell and the pattern of the seeds on sunflowers.

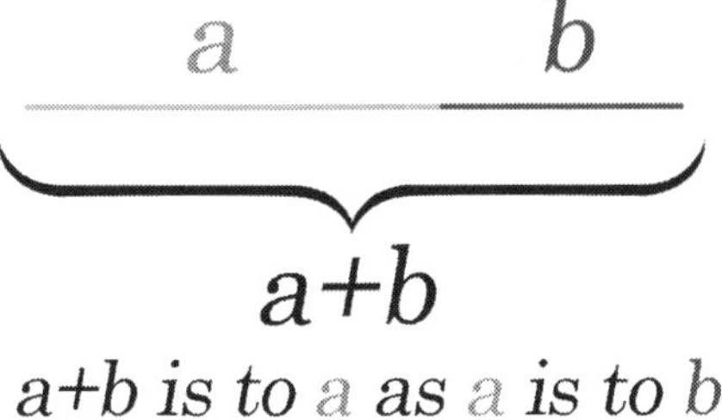

Formula for the golden ratio.

One of the most important elements in creating beautiful art is composition. Balance and proportion are critical to creating a successful masterpiece, working both with color and proportion. This formula has been used in masterpieces by world-renowned artists such as Leonardo da Vinci, Michelangelo, and Rembrandt. It has also been used in ancient architecture such as the Great Pyramids, the Parthenon, and the Cathedral of Chartres. Most importantly, the golden ratio was used in creating the greatest masterpiece and architecture of all: the human body. If you know what to look for, you will start to see these patterns.

You may notice examples of the golden ratio in the human face:

- Length of face to the width of face
- Distance between the lips and where the eyebrows meet to the length of nose
- Length of face to the distance between tip of jaw and where the eyebrows meet
- Length of mouth to the width of nose
- Width of nose to the distance between nostrils
- Distance between pupils to the distance between eyebrows

People are attracted to other people who exhibit balance and harmony in their appearance. Human faces and bodies that most people consider as beautiful possess these dimensions falling within the golden ratio. We are subconsciously programmed to pick up on this symmetry and balance.

Figures that we view as having good proportions are seen as desirable because they fall within the golden ratio. We subconsciously notice the golden ratio when we recognize that something looks good; however, most of us don't know the science behind why this is appealing to us. The ideal body proportions, from our teeth to our toes, fall within this formula.

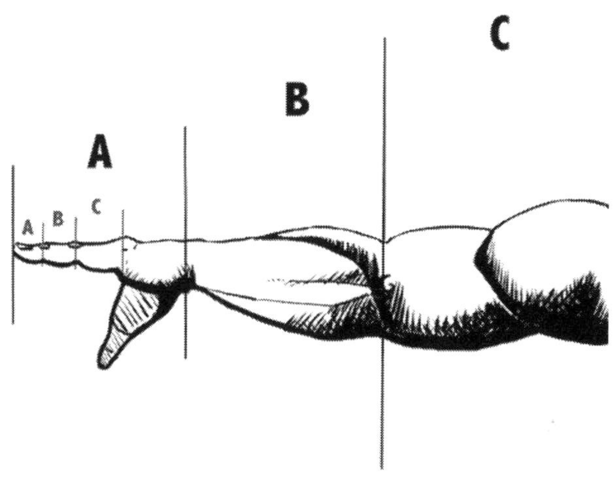

Notice the golden ratio proportion of the arm to the elbow to the wrist.*

You may notice examples of the golden ratio in the human body:

- The distance between the fingertip and the elbow to the distance between the wrist and the elbow
- The distance between the shoulder line and the top of the head to the head length
- The distance between the navel and the top of the head to the distance between the shoulder line and the top of the head
- The distance between the navel and knee to the distance between the knee and the end of the foot

*(golden ratio body proportions from *http://betterbodyguide.com*)

YOU ARE A MASTERPIECE

The good news is that you are not expected to be perfect. No one fits into the golden ratio perfectly, and if we were all clones walking around with the same features, the world would be a boring place. Imperfections add individuality and personality to you that are uniquely yours.

Methods of measurement aren't meant to limit us from developing our own vision for our own beauty. The DRES System is not intended to hold you back in any way or to place you into a box. Simplification of complex concepts have been distilled to make the system easy to use. It's meant to give you an idea of where you are so that we can add balance and harmony to your proportions.

DRES System Personal Stylists are taught to value the uniqueness of each individual; we want to help each client tap into the power of attraction that is a fundamental instinct in all of us. Once you have a clear idea of where you are and where you want to go, anything is possible.

Remember it's all about achieving excellence, not perfection. Perfection is unobtainable, and pursuing it can lead to obsessive behaviors. Excellence is when you have reached your full potential.

Think of yourself as a blank canvas every day: a clean, crisp, untouched surface with never-ending potential. The possibilities are endless. When you make clothing selections, you are essentially creating art. Paint with the colors of the fabrics. Draw with lines that are created by the shapes of the apparel. Sculpt a new silhouette with your outfit.

- **Painting** = colors in your personal palette
- **Drawing** = lines in your clothing
- **Sculpting** = shapes in your silhouette

Canvases come in many shapes and sizes and it can be difficult to know where to start. You have the potential to be a masterpiece every day with the support from a DRES System–Certified Personal Stylist, who can help you curate a successful wardrobe that brings out the best in you.

CREATION OF A STYLING SYSTEM

I created the DRES System and began training certified personal stylists to help women get the tools and support they need to build a wardrobe and feel like a masterpiece. In creating the DRES System, I drew from my background as a lifelong artist and painter, my aesthetics training in beauty school, lessons learned while obtaining my degree in visual communications, and my analytical nature. Many of the techniques we use in the DRES System are based on painting techniques, design principles, and color theory.

The DRES System takes styling to a whole new level with the use of science. After analyzing hundreds of body shapes, I came up with a math-based formula to identify my clients' dominant body shapes. I chose to identify these body shapes as the precious gems: Diamond, Ruby, Emerald, Sapphire (DRES) to instill value, self-worth, and pride in the uniqueness of every figure, and to ease the stress of dressing. Our core belief is that every woman is a precious gem and no matter what your body shape, size, or age, there is beauty within you just waiting to be revealed.

In addition to the body shape assessment formula, I also created a formula for assessing body proportions and face shapes. Because I wanted a complete system, I developed a personalized color assessment process, wardrobe editing method, and personal shopping techniques. With all this valuable information, dressing becomes easier. Once you understand both your body shape and proportions, you are empowered to make wiser purchasing decisions.

Knowledge & Clarity > Wise Choices > Saving $$$ > Power

Consider all the clothes in your closet that you do not wear. Typically, we estimate that most people wear only 15 percent of what's in their wardrobe. Think about this for a moment. Let's say the total value of your wardrobe is $10,000. If you wear only 15 percent of it, that's $8,500 of wasted time, money, and effort. Not to mention it's taking up a lot of space in your closet and adding confusion to your morning dressing routine. You deserve better!

DRES SYSTEM PROFILE

"I've read countless books and articles about dressing for your body shape, but none of them compare to the way you've broken it down with actual measurements—now I know for certain that my torso is shorter than average. When I saw labels I already love, I knew you guys were on to something!"
—Candice Caldwell (Founder of Fashion Ethic, online boutique)

DRES Body Shapes

Getting dressed is not easy for everyone: you are not wearing 85 percent of your wardrobe and appearance can be a very emotional issue. Our DRES Personal Stylists are dedicated to improving the way women see their bodies and providing the highest-quality services and tools to help them look and feel beautiful and confident.

The reason this proven system works is because its simplicity brings clarity, and our unique personalized techniques customize it for *you*. Our goal is to provide you with the tools and support you need to curate a wardrobe that reflects your lifestyle. We want you to stand out as the unique individual that you are.

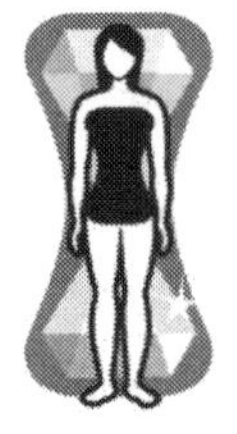
diamond

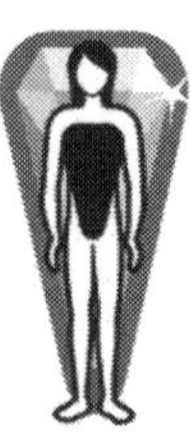
ruby

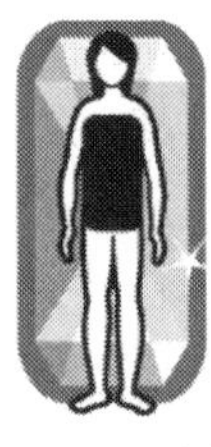
emerald

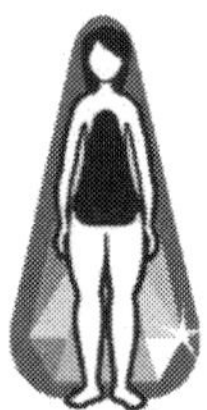
sapphire

Diamond: The beauty of the diamond body shape is in the symmetry of the shoulders and hips. While you are starting out with a beautifully balanced body, you could lose this symmetry quickly with the wrong clothing and accessory choices. Look to widen the shoulders a little, and show off your waist.

Ruby: The beauty of the ruby body shape is in the slender hips and thighs. You either have a large bustline or broad shoulders. Create symmetry and balance in your shape with the right clothing and accessory choices. Look to reduce the chest and/or shoulder area, and show off your legs.

Emerald: The beauty of the emerald body shape is in the symmetry of the shoulders and hips. Your arms and legs are proportionate to the rest of your body. You could lose this symmetry quickly with the wrong clothing and accessory choices. Look to slim the waist, and reveal your assets.

Sapphire: The beauty of the sapphire body shape is in the slender arms and small rib cage. Your décolleté begs to be highlighted. Create symmetry and balance in your shape with the right clothing and accessory choices. Look to reduce the width of the hips and thigh area, and show off your waist and arms.

DRES Face Shapes

People are often confused by which face shape they have. To make this easy we have developed a math-based formula for determining your facial shape. This tells us if your face most resembles a Diamond, Ruby, Emerald, or Sapphire and if it is long, average, or short. To learn more about the DRES System face shapes, see chapter 7 on Face Styling.

DRES Fashion Styles

The five fashion styles defined for the DRES System will help you create a refined image and reflect the image you intend to project.

Your fashion style should first be authentic, by aligning with your personality type. Second, it should be appropriate for the activity or event you are planning for. Classic, chic, romantic, ethnic, and dramatic are the five fashion styles we use in the DRES System. Everyone has one fashion style that is most dominant. Can you easily identify yours? One of our personal stylists can assess your body shape and show you how to style it!

- **Classic:** gracious, refined, and sophisticated
- **Chic:** modern, self-assured, and sharp
- **Romantic:** friendly, casual, and whimsical
- **Ethnic:** diverse, authentic, and cultural
- **Dramatic:** energetic, exciting, and strong

DRES Color Palette

Professional personal color analysis is one of the most valuable services you can receive that will help you for years to come. Simply wearing the right colors can make a huge difference in how you look and feel, and save you time shopping, too. Your DRES System–Certified Personal Stylist can define your forty-two Ultimate Colors out of over five hundred possibilities. We use our exclusive DRES System to provide a detailed analysis of your individual coloring and create a personalized Color Palette, with beautiful fabric swatches, made just for you.

We also offer twelve different prepared color identification sets with thirty-six fabric swatches. These are very helpful if you already know your color range.

WHAT'S YOUR DRES CODE?

"I like that the DRES System has simplified terminology, so I did not have to figure out if the clothes were meant for me."
—Jody Hurd, Client SD2 (Sapphire, Dramatic, Color Code 2)

The DRES Code is simply your Personal DRES Profile turned into a three-character set. It is a code that tells you if an item will work for you.

Narrowing down the options and cutting the time it takes to locate the perfect item for you, the code has three elements:

- Body Shape
- Fashion Style
- Color Code

This is an easy way to know if an item is going to work for your personal style before even trying it on, taking some of the guesswork out of shopping. For example, if this is your DRES Profile:

- Body Shape: Ruby
- Fashion Style: Chic
- Color Range: 8

Then this would be your DRES Code: RC8.

Not everyone fits nicely into just one area. Many people may be a combination of these; however, to make it easier, we would use your dominant body shape, fashion style, and color range to devise your DRES Code.

USING A PERSONAL STYLIST IS POWERFUL

"I'm a bookkeeper, so I'm not great with anything artistic, including dressing myself. Margaret was able to come into my home and, in three visits, I had a different view and a more positive outlook. It even inspired me to go on a diet, and I've lost 30 pounds so far! The experience was a little scary, but I was made comfortable by Margaret's calm, reassuring manner and relaxed approach to the DRES System. I now go into my closet and am better able to pick out what to wear without it causing me anxiety or stress."

—Linda Cavanaugh, Client SR7 (Sapphire, Romantic, Color Code 7)

Everyone could use a personal stylist. I believe that, someday soon, this will become as common as having a hairstylist. It's hard for us to see ourselves in an objective way. Even when we look in the mirror, we don't see what others do. We tend to look at ourselves with bias; first checking out our problem areas, and then completely overlooking our best features and our overall image.

A DRES System Personal Stylist will get to know your personality and preferences though supportive, private, and inspiring one-on-one consultations. There's no judgment—we're here to help! In the training to become a DRES System–Certified Personal Stylist (DRES Stylist), we teach techniques on how to empower our clients with excellent knowledge about their appearance, and we also talk in great detail about the customer experience when working with a DRES Stylist. All information shared in our private consulting appointments is confidential; we never disclose who we are working with. When you leave your consulting appointment, you will have a heightened sense of confidence and feel more self-assured in how you present yourself.

One of the greatest gifts is having someone beside you, giving you permission to do what you deep down already want to do, but, for whatever reason, haven't been able to act on. This reminds me of a client I once worked with. She was a mother of two grown teenagers, and she lived in a beautiful home in a nice part of town. When she greeted me at the door, she was wearing a plain, solid-colored T-shirt and baggy sweats. Her hair was unstyled, and she wore no makeup. As I entered her home, I was taken aback by how expertly it was decorated. It was so beautifully designed, it could have been featured in *ELLE DECOR* magazine. I could not take in enough of the details of each room as we quickly passed them, heading to the dining room, where we would start her personal profile assessment. Later when we made our way upstairs to her bedroom to view her wardrobe, we passed all of the other rooms in the home, decorated with just as much skill and grace.

I finally shared with her how fond I was of her home and asked if she decorated it herself or if she had some help. I was amazed to learn that she did this all on her own. It quickly became clear to me that this woman poured all of herself into her family and home and did not reserve anything for herself. Her home was ornate and well loved with lots of color, fabrics, accessories, and family photos. In contrast, her personal image was communicating plain, unimaginative, and neglected. I could tell she had a lot of work to do on the inside to get her to take as much pride in her appearance as she had in her home.

Too often we see that women have put the needs of their families or careers before themselves. What women fail to understand is that people will treat you as well as you treat yourself. When I am confronted with excuses such as "I don't have enough time in the day" or "I want to wait till I lose some weight," I say, "Don't put yourself on hold!" Start treating yourself well today and everything else will fall into place.

It's priceless to know someone who will give you honest feedback and is not swayed by making a sale, as is the case with many free styling services in department stores. DRES Stylists are not locked into one brand. We search all stores and brands to bring you the best fit for your needs. Imagine having someone who has your best interests in mind and has taken the time to listen, non-critically assess, and understand you. A professional who can take into consideration your existing clothing pieces and help you build a well-rounded wardrobe over time that fits your DRES Profile and lifestyle. It's like having an objective and professionally trained shopping buddy!

Polished Presence

A personal stylist helps you to have a polished presence for all those important occasions. Sometimes it's not so much about *what* you wear as *how* you wear it. A personal stylist can help you curate key pieces in your wardrobe and assemble complete outfits documented in your personalized look book. No more walking into your closet full of clothes and feeling like you have nothing to wear. You will be prepared for any occasion.

One of the best parts about working with a personal stylist is that they help you step outside of your comfort zone and try new things. We often hear, "Wow, I would never have thought that would look good on me." You may have items in your wardrobe that you have never worn together and a stylist can give you a whole new perspective on new ensembles and inspire you to try new things.

Empowered Clarity

As we move though life, sometimes our fashion style gets stuck. You may feel you lack a vision for your personal style. A personal stylist can help you stay updated each season without falling victim to the current trends that are not appropriate for your unique profile. A solid understanding of your style will make you look confident and effortlessly chic. Working with a personal stylist can keep your look fresh, polished, and current.

Ten Reasons to Hire a Personal Stylist

1. Discover your beauty inside and out.
2. Save time and money on misguided purchases.
3. Find what fits quickly and effortlessly.
4. Build confidence.
5. Learn to do more with less.
6. Refine your image.
7. Get a fresh perspective.
8. Define colors and fashion style.
9. Understand body shape and proportions.
10. Know what to wear and when.

Once you know more, you can do better. Understanding and defining your shape's unique proportions, your unique coloring, and style loves will give you empowered clarity. With this newfound clarity, you will be able to achieve the image you desire because knowledge is power.

THE WARDROBE YOU CRAVE

"Before the DRES System, when I had to decide what to wear each day, I was stressed. Now it is a breeze! I can just look at the pictures. I feel better when I step out and know that my clothes make me look great. The DRES System has really given my confidence a boost."
—Susan Coon, Client DC11 (Diamond, Chic, Color Code 11)

There are some moments in life that stick in our memories forever. For me it was standing in line in the school yard during first grade. The bell had just rung, and we were lining up to go into class. There was a girl in front of me who had long, perfectly straight, golden hair; a dress that looked as if it was freshly pressed; neatly folded over, white knee-high socks; and new patent leather shoes. Clearly, she had a mother who knew a thing or two about style and took great care of her daughter. All I could think about in that moment was I wanted to be *that girl*.

Have You Ever Wanted to Be "That Girl"?

- The one who always looks polished and pulled together, right down to her perfect pedicure!
- The one who wears the most appropriate outfit for every occasion.
- The one who is always wearing the most current fashions and radiates confidence.

Imagine:

- Having a wardrobe full of clothes that you love!
- Feeling confident and happy when you look in the mirror.
- Having the perfect outfit for every occasion.

You can be "that girl" at work or play. Getting dressed for the office or social gatherings should not be stressful. With a well-laid-out wardrobe plan and a clear understanding of what works for your shape, coloring, and style, you can achieve the image you desire.

Live for today, and don't put yourself on hold. We often hear women say, "I would love to work on my wardrobe once I lose some weight." Please don't be one of these women. This is self-punishment, and none of us feels motivated to change when we feel punished.

The idea is to treat yourself well. Work on enhancing your image, and you will start to receive compliments. This is exactly the encouragement you need to keep going. Once you are focused on treating yourself well and are happy with yourself, it will be much easier to start focusing on weight loss. In fact, most women look twenty to fifty pounds lighter after working with a stylist who can help with the proper fit and teach illusion dressing. These are the kinds of immediate results that we are all looking for.

Now that you have had an overview of all the components that make up the DRES System, the following is a collection of different perspectives on psychology, trends, style, editing, accessories, face styling, makeup, and being timeless, written by some of our top DRES System–Certified Personal Stylists, who want to share with you tips on tapping into your image power, reaching your full potential, and giving yourself permission to be your best.

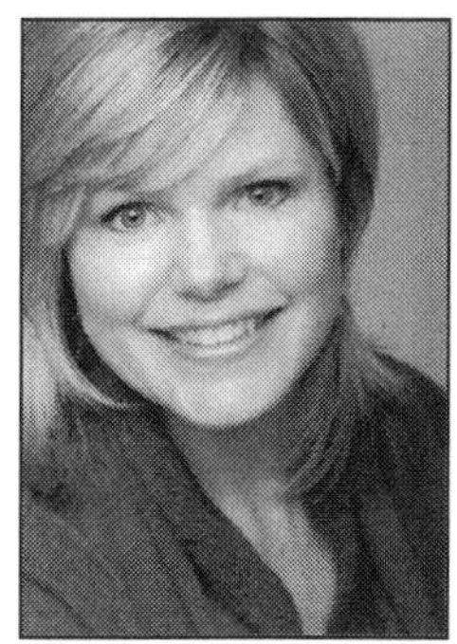

Margaret Spencer

Founder and DRES System Personal Stylist

DRES System
www.DRESsystem.com
ms@DRESsystem.com
Seattle, Washington

Margaret has always been attracted to the beauty found in the world and the people within it. During high school, Margaret attended beauty school to become an aesthetician and began her own business providing in-home manicures and sculpted nails at the age of eighteen. This would be the first go in her lifelong pursuit of entrepreneurship, a path she chose due to her desire to build something that would make a positive difference.

After studying visual communications at the Art Institute of Seattle, she continued with her passion for business and design by building a graphic design company that she successfully ran for fifteen years. Looking for a change of pace, she then founded a drop-in art studio and school where she taught people how anyone could be an artist.

Now Margaret focuses her creative energy, eye for design, and entrepreneurial drive on growing and sharing the power of the DRES System. Taking from all her past experiences, she set out to give women the right tools and support to instill self-worth and acceptance of their bodies. She knows firsthand how women can struggle with how to dress their figures and feel confident in their individual images.

In between consulting with clients and traveling the country to teach stylist-training classes, Margaret loves predicting the latest trends, impressionistic painting, and playing with her very fluffy yet tough, Miniature Goldendoodle, Steve. Along with her dog, Margaret also lives with a loving husband and two daughters in Seattle, Washington.

"I wish for you what I wish for myself—the opportunities to reach your fullest potential."

CHAPTER 2

PSYCHOLOGY

Our Relationship With Clothes

By Corey Urbina

Ever since childhood, I have been a people-watcher. Even though the adults in my life gently reminded me that staring was impolite, I just couldn't help myself. Little did they know this curious habit of mine would one day serve me well in my career as a personal stylist.

People fascinate me. My idea of a perfect day includes sitting at a sidewalk café, soaking in the somatic and sartorial landscape. I first study people's clothing and take in the colors, styles, and fabrics they wear. I also look at how individuals assemble their clothing and accessories into a unified collage. Each person, from the style-challenged to the style superstar, teaches me something new.

Although manner of dress first captures my interest, curiosity about what lies beneath someone's exterior holds my attention. In my mind, as I attempt to read individuals, I wonder about their psychological makeup and imagine what kind of lives they lead. People reveal clues to their stories without ever uttering a word. They speak volumes about who they are by what they wear, how they stand, and by their facial expressions and gestures. Some individuals glide gracefully as they walk, while others slump and slouch. Their eyes sometimes express sadness. A person's staccato movements expose their anxiety. All of us constantly transmit messages about ourselves that others receive and interpret. Everything we notice about an individual, from a shrug of the shoulders to the paisley pattern in a flowing neck scarf, provides us with clues about the person within.

The inconsistencies in a person's appearance also spark my curiosity. I notice when clothing and body language send conflicting messages, and my mind immediately imagines the reasons for these image incongruities. On one of my recent trips from Washington, D.C., to Greenville, South Carolina, I spent a few extra hours at Reagan National Airport. As I waited for my flight, I noticed a man in his early twenties wearing low-slung, cut-off sweatpants, a rumpled shirt, and white athletic socks with shower shoes. He kept hiking up his pants to prevent them from sliding past his hips and falling to the floor. By today's style standards, nothing about his attire seemed out of the ordinary except for the two pieces of Louis Vuitton luggage he toted. The person seated next to me also noticed this apparition and quipped, "We all know what this guy's parents just gave him for graduation."

I spent the remainder of my wait pondering why this person's luggage taste differed so drastically from his personal style. I would have expected him to throw his belongings in a beat-up duffel bag. Instead, he not only opted for Louis Vuitton suitcases costing close to $4,000 but also chose this designer's most conspicuously expensive *LV* signature pattern. Material like this makes me want to write a novel. It would explore the life of a rich but rebellious youth who struggles between opposing worlds to figure out where he belongs. Since appearances only give us pieces of the puzzle, I'll never know this traveler's real story.

Much of our understanding on the role of nonverbal behavior in communication comes from the pioneering research of UCLA professor Albert Mehrabian. His study dealt with how individuals process and respond to messages involving feelings and emotions during conversation. According to Mehrabian, "when an incongruity exists between the spoken word and how you deliver it, 7 percent of the message is conveyed through your words, 38 percent is revealed through your vocal quality and a whopping 55 percent of your message comes through your gestures, expression and posture" (*Body Language for Dummies*, Elizabeth Kuhnke, 2012).

Although Mehrabian's findings only relate to communication concerning feelings and emotions, they illustrate the significance of words, tone of voice, and body language in communication. Mehrabian's research has enormous significance for stylists because our work centers upon a critical component of nonverbal communication: appearance. We teach clients how to present an image that captures their strengths and positively affects others. For self-concept develops not only from an individual's self perceptions but also from how others perceive them and respond to them. An individual internalizes cues from others, and this feedback either bolsters self-concept—or diminishes it. This phenomenon is known as the "looking-glass self" (*Human Nature and the Social Order*, Charles Horton Cooley, 1902). I dress clients for success in life because I want them to project self-confidence and self-esteem and to internalize these qualities. The DRES System provides the perfect framework for individuals to move toward self-awareness, self-acceptance, and confidence. In my experience, clients often view the styling process as one component of a broader self-development effort. They welcome honest and constructive feedback on how to reach their full style potential. We personal stylists assess each individual's unique styling needs and help them to identify and achieve desired goals through a step-by-step process of education and support. The result is nothing short of amazing.

"Everyone possesses their own unique beauty and authentic style. It's our job to bring out that beauty for the world to see" (*DRES System Personal Stylist Training Manual,* Margaret Spencer, 2008). We take the transformative journey with our clients and witness from a front-row seat the positive results that take place both on the outside and inside. Nothing compares to the feeling of knowing that we played a part in changing lives.

I also feel privileged to share milestones in clients' lives right along with them. I'm there when a client picks out her first professional suit, clothes for an anniversary cruise, or her mother-of-the-bride dress.

People change their lives every day. I met one of my clients, Vanessa, at a critical point in her life. Vanessa's recent marriage, coupled with the rapid growth of her business, provided the catalyst to lose weight, get fit, and enhance her image. Meeting me gave Vanessa the extra nudge she needed to pursue all of these goals. With each step in the program, she shed her insecurities and met every challenge with single-minded determination. Vanessa emerged from this process feeling reborn and looking stunning. She expressed her appreciation for my work by saying, "I can't tell you how life changing this whole process is for me." How many of us get to hear those words in the course of a day?

All positive change requires self-awareness and commitment. No one hires a stylist unless they are ready to make an investment in themselves. For some, the prospect of opening their closet and their lives to a stranger is scary. Our work sometimes involves changing habits and deeply ingrained personal beliefs. Those who do take the step to enhance their style approach the process with enthusiasm and openness. The size of the steps depends on a number of factors including self-concept, personality, life circumstances, and style goals.

RELATIONSHIPS MATTER

The client-stylist relationship forms the foundation for a successful styling experience. The personal stylist's job requires that we read people well and build their trust. I rely on my counseling training every day in my work with clients. I meet them wherever they are on the style spectrum and in life, and tailor an approach that fully engages them. My methodologies vary from client to client. I may ask clients to look through magazines or fabric swatches to identify styles and colors that please them. Sometimes I'll ask them to describe their most favorite dress growing up or a time in their life when they felt the most stylish. If I sense that clients seem uncomfortable answering certain questions, I switch gears.

Dealing with personal and sensitive topics such as body image sometimes stirs clients' emotions. They may express frustration that few items in their closet fit them well because of a recent weight gain. DRES System Personal Stylists pick up on these feelings and know how to diffuse them. Facing the three-way, full-length mirrors and fluorescent lighting of store dressing rooms can dampen the spirits of even the most self-assured among us. To ward off occasional dressing room doldrums, I sometimes suggest a break for coffee or lunch. I use this time to talk about how the shopping experience illuminated my understanding of the client's style profile.

WHO HIRES A PERSONAL STYLIST?

One of the first questions people ask when they hear about what I do for a living is, "Who is your typical client?" In reviewing my client list, I came up with this system of classification that takes into account most of the reasons why women hire a personal stylist:

The Overextended

These are the "I try to do it all" folks. Women in this group work, raise children, manage households, go to soccer games, hold office in the P.T.A., take spinning class, volunteer in the community, and try to maintain some semblance of sanity. To say they are stretched thin doesn't even come close to describing their lives.

Sarah Jessica Parker portrays the character of Kate Reddy in the movie *I Don't Know How She Does It.* She plays a multitasking, list-making supermom and business executive. A successful investment manager, Kate is constantly packing and unpacking from business trips and pulls off the impossible on minimal sleep. At night, instead of counting sheep, she stares at the ceiling composing her to-do lists. She leads a frantic, rat-race life and takes little time for herself. The Kates in my life have me on speed dial. They need me to organize their closets, shop for them each season, and assemble all of their go-to outfits for them. Since everything else in their lives requires juggling and multitasking, they need style to be simple.

The Strategists

These women always look at the big picture; they think analytically and maintain a decade-at-a-glance appointment book. They regularly set goals, and keep their closets and their finances organized. Procrastination is a dirty word to these folks. They know their style, and have determined a clothing budget even before I step through the front door. Although their closets are uncluttered, we spend time analyzing the pros and cons of each item of clothing they own. Strategists hire me because they value my expertise and know that I will help them make wise clothing choices. They trust me to shop for them and expect that I will find quality items at the best prices.

The Voyagers

A specific life event or a series of occurrences attracts these women to my business. My dear friend and client Lynn decided to treat herself to a stylist for her sixty-fifth birthday. Having scrimped on her wardrobe for most of her life, she decided to invest in new clothes. Although she always looked chic wearing consignment and thrift store finds, this time she decided to drop some cash on core wardrobe pieces. First, she and I weeded out the undesirables from her closet. Then, off we went to high-end stores like Saks Fifth Avenue and Neiman Marcus. The result was a restocked closet containing several classy items.

Another client and her husband boldly left their jobs, sold their home, and moved with their two young children from upstate New York to Greenville, South Carolina. Within a span of six months, they settled into a new life. The couple moved from an apartment into a new home, enrolled their children in preschool, and started working in their new jobs. Before leaving New York, my client chucked most of her wardrobe. I shopped fast and furiously to ensure that she had enough clothes to last her a few months. A year later, I am still fine-tuning her wardrobe.

For other Voyagers, the catalyst for change may be a promotion, retirement, childbirth, or divorce. Emotions run the spectrum from exhilaration to grief. The common denominator in all these scenarios is change coupled with a desire for renewal. I love working with individuals in this group because they inspire me with their resiliency and optimism.

Voyagers see challenges as opportunities for reinvention. Their attitudes remind me of this quote by writer Maria Robinson: "Nobody can go back and start a new beginning, but anyone can start today and make a new ending."

THE ORIGINS OF PERSONAL STYLE

"Know first, who you are; and then adorn yourself accordingly"
—Epictetus, *Discourses*, 3.1

Merriam-Webster's Dictionary defines style as "a quality of imagination and individuality expressed in one's actions and tastes." Clients often tell me that they either lack style, or they describe their style as dowdy and frumpy. They usually appear shocked when I tell them that everyone possesses style whether they know it or not. In one of my blog pieces, "How to Tap into Your Personal Style" (www.stylemattersgreenville.com/how-to-tap-into-your-personal-style/), I write that style "incubates in our self-conscious and emerges under the right conditions."

DRES System Personal Stylists create the "right conditions" for clients to gain style clarity. This revelation takes place during the client profile. The fashion style quiz, a pivotal exercise in this introductory session, serves two important purposes: it clearly establishes the fact that authentic style originates from within and that it influences our fashion choices.

Because so many women let fashion trends dictate what they wear, they have never given much thought to the concept of style identity. Without this anchor, individuals stay stuck in style limbo. They wander aimlessly through the vast recesses of a mall, wasting an abundance of time and money on the wrong clothing purchases. I can't tell you how often I've heard this woeful refrain during a closet edit: "I don't know why I bought this. It just isn't me."

Those who seek to express themselves fully through style spend time in self-reflection. Every personal quality and life experience contributes to the development of style. Genuine style also communicates one's goals and aspirations. Those on a fast track to a corporate partnership make vastly different clothing choices than individuals who seek a nontraditional career trajectory.

Once a client is encouraged to delve into their style, they begin to remember what factors influenced their style development. One of my clients grew up in a family of limited means. She didn't have many clothes as a child, and her mother took her shopping only for necessities. Consequently, her fashion vocabulary remained underdeveloped. Into her adulthood, she carried the belief that clothes were for function and not fashion. She didn't entertain many thoughts about what she liked and how she wanted to look. She also felt guilty when she bought clothes that weren't on sale. The fashion style quiz gave her permission to explore a part of herself that she didn't know existed. I strongly believe in the work that we do as stylists because it helps people uncover who they are. It is no coincidence that my twitter name is @wearwhoyouare.

In spite of the fact that everyone expresses their own unique style brand, definite style similarities exist among individuals. The DRES System has examined all of the fashion styles and distilled them down to five categories. Here is an opportunity to step into another's clothes and try on their style personality. Hopefully, these vignettes will give you a glimpse of the psychology of what we wear.

FIVE STYLE PERSONALITIES, PERSONIFIED

Claire the Classic

Claire describes herself as serious and practical. She works in the banking industry and hopes to advance quickly within her company. She has a degree in finance and plans to pursue graduate studies at night. Because

Claire budgets her money carefully, she hopes to buy a home in two years. Claire's classic tastes have remained constant since they emerged during early adolescence. Her wardrobe reflects her conservative and pragmatic tendencies. She wears tailored pieces with simple lines. She gravitates toward solids and neutrals that reflect her profession's dress preferences as well as her reserved nature. Her minimal jewelry and accessory choices make a quiet statement. Guided by her budget-conscious inclinations, Claire buys high-quality items with long style lives. What's in her closet? A tailored, no-iron blouse and blue blazer from J.Crew. Adjectives that describe Claire: practical, trustworthy, hardworking.

Carly the Chic

Carly lives in New York City and owns her own website design company. In her spare time, she makes presentations to community groups on social media marketing strategies. Carly believes in staying current with the latest social and fashion trends. Wherever she goes, she looks sophisticated and polished. She reads *InStyle* and *Lucky* each month and follows fashion blogs. Others defer to her for fashion advice. Color, contemporary designs, and interesting details distinguish her closet from others. Carly invests time and money on her clothes, hair, makeup, and nails. What's in Carly's closet? A black, three-quarter-length ruched sleeve, shrunken blazer and python print pencil skirt by BCBG. Adjectives that describe Carly: modern, edgy, energetic.

Raquel the Romantic

Raquel gravitates toward feminine styles that grace her curves. A self-described "girly girl," she loves soft, flowing fabrics; ruffles; pleating; and dresses with waists. Her idea of a great dress showcases her décolleté and waistline. She loves floral prints, pastels, chiffons, and velvets. Raquel adores being a mom and nesting at home. She maintains close relationships with a few girlfriends and regularly socializes with them. After putting her children to bed in the evenings, she spends relaxing time with her husband. What's in Raquel's closet? Coldwater Creek gathered chiffon skirt with asymmetrical hem and ruffle-front blouse. Adjectives to describe Raquel: whimsical, feminine, fun.

Elly the Ethnic

Elly's clothing represents her expansive worldview. She reads a great deal about the history and traditions of other cultures and travels extensively. She has a curious nature and fully embraces life each day. Elly begins each morning with meditation and yoga practice. Her concern for preserving the environment prompts her to wear mostly natural and eco-friendly fabrics. She volunteers at a local food co-op and also initiated a recycling program at her apartment complex. Elly stands out in her wide-legged linen trousers, thrift store finds, and natural gemstone and beaded jewelry. Elly usually decorates her wrists with assorted bracelets and wears wide-brimmed hats. It's no surprise that Elly is enamored with the fashions of the 1960s. What's in Elly's closet? An Anthropologie embroidered tunic, Tom's ballet slippers, and silver and turquoise jewelry by Silpada. Adjectives to describe Elly: nonconformist, earthy, eco-conscious.

Dana the Dramatic

Dana is a daring extravert with oodles of charisma. She enjoys turning heads when she walks into a room and, boy! Can she work a room. She is an idea person with boundless creative energy. Dana looks for clothes matching her personal power and thrives on combining unexpected colors, fabrics, and patterns. She dares to be different by wearing the newest, most edgy designs. To Dana, the world is truly a stage, so many of her pieces resemble costumes. Each item is carefully chosen for its wow factor. What's in her closet? A black, mid-length coat dress, trimmed in red, with dolman sleeves and shoulder epaulets, made by an indie designer. Adjectives to describe Dana: risk-taker, unorthodox, intense.

The work of DRES System Personal Stylists relative to style identity sometimes completely illuminates self-perceptions. One of my clients conducts corporate training programs designed to improve workplace culture by focusing on communication, problem solving, and team building. Her work is cutting-edge and experimental. She acts not only as a facilitator but as a coach during these training sessions.

When I initially met with her, she expressed some ambivalence about her conservative professional style. She felt her image lacked a certain something, but she didn't know exactly what. Her uniform for her trainings consisted of two-piece suits or neutral separates. The fashion style quiz revealed her as a classic dresser, with strong romantic tendencies. As she disclosed more about her work, it became apparent that she used her dynamic personality and her skills to engage and inspire people. Two key ingredients in the training involved building trust and having fun. Both of us realized that her work would benefit if she brought out the whimsical and playful side of her style personality in the way that she dressed. This revelation framed the rest of our work together. During her closet edit, I demonstrated how she could add whimsy to her wardrobe by decoupling suits and creatively mixing and matching separates. I showed her how to weave in her favorite leather jacket and lace blouse by pairing them with her suit bottoms. I also demonstrated techniques for using color and accessories to liven up her look. In the end, my client projected an image more closely aligned with her personality and professional brand.

Even though other clients might not experience quite so remarkable an aha moment, they benefit in other important ways from taking the fashion style quiz. Learning about their multifaceted style personalities often gives clients permission to explore their more dormant fashion instincts. This exploration often leads to their willingness to literally try on different styles to see how they look and feel in them. Clients may also blend their styles to create a signature style. By taking these style-defining steps, clients reframe their perceptions of who they are and how they want others to perceive them. If the fashion quiz conforms closely to an individual's self-concept of style, the results give them the confidence that they need to stay grounded in their style.

Once clients gain style clarity, they move on to the next step, which involves some deeper self-reflection. Clients are asked to articulate their physical and personal strengths, an exercise that many find challenging. To encourage clients, I ask them to think back on all of the qualities that have helped them accomplish goals, deal with adversity, and manage day-to-day responsibilities successfully. Throughout the styling process, I remind clients of their external and internal assets, and I repeatedly use the same words that they have chosen to describe themselves. At the conclusion of our work together, most of my clients confidently add to their list of assets.

WHAT INFLUENCES STYLE EXPRESSION?

Although many women adhere to one dominant style, more often than not they see themselves as style hybrids. Which style emerges on any given day depends on several factors: their assessment of what's appropriate for a situation, how they want to be perceived, and their mood. For example, a normally classic dresser may buy a floral instead of a solid top and a pair of bright green (rather than khaki) capris for a cruise to the Caribbean. A chic dresser who loves always being on trend may wear a navy or gray Theory suit for a crucial business meeting. Of course, this practice takes style intelligence or the ability to make smart choices about what and what not to wear for each situation.

D.C. fashion blogger Alison Gary often writes about the connection between mood and fashion. In a recent posting entitled "Black Is My Mood and My Dress" (http://www.wardrobeoxygen.com), Alison described how she went through the contents of her closet to find an outfit that fit her tired and glum mood. She passed over the items that looked "too cheery" and decided on a black dress, black shoes, and black jewelry. By shrouding herself in black, Alison needed to unequivocally express her dark mood.

To illustrate the relationship between style and mood, just consider the angst that many women go through when packing for a trip. Some women I know would rather have a root canal than face this dreaded task. Most of my clients admit that they end up bringing far more clothes than they actually need. The experience of schlepping heavy suitcases around while on holiday doesn't usually deter them from overpacking the next time. One of the women in my book club summed up the packing conundrum. She said she needed a variety of clothing options because "I never know how I'm going to feel." This comment raises the notion that we not only need to express ourselves through clothing but also seek congruency between our appearance and our feelings. Without the proper clothes, an experience is missing an important synapse that allows for full self-expression.

Having spent a summer off from college traveling around Europe with only a small weekender for all of my belongings, I can attest to the strangeness of that experience. I essentially wore the same four outfits every day for the entire time I worked as an au pair in London and traveled around Spain and France with girlfriends. The experience was akin to *Invasion of the Body Snatchers*. I did not feel completely like me, nor did I particularly enjoy looking at myself in the mirror day after day in the same clothes. I also mourned the loss of my favorite daily creative exercise: dressing. To add some variety to my appearance, I walked into a beauty salon in Paris with waist-length hair and came out with a 1970s Jane Fonda shag hairdo. On the flight back home from Europe, I fantasized about how I would destroy my travel clothes when I got home. Would I burn them? Cut them up in a million tiny pieces, and *then* burn them? In the end I delighted in heaving them into the trash.

I now advise people on how and what to pack for trips, using the DRES System capsule wardrobe approach. I also ask clients to select their favorite color as well as accessories and two outfits that epitomize their persona. If a client loves turquoise, I suggest that she purchase items in this palette such as a scarf, belt, cropped cardigan, ballet flats, earrings, and bracelets that she could easily tuck into a suitcase. If possible, we try to work with both of the client's outfit selections. Creatively changing up accessories and shoes breathes new life into core pieces and adds to their versatility. Clients thank me when they open up their suitcase and see color and friendly clothes instead of a sea of sensible, black travel separates.

I think that the desire for a wardrobe repertoire when away from home runs deeper than the need for self-expression. Clothes provide comfort and variety, but they also validate the fact that you remain the same person wherever you go. My mother spent almost four years in Europe and the Middle East during World War II as a U.S. Army nurse. She had striking good looks and fantastic style. Only she could look like a runway model in photos while she posed in front of a tent hospital at the North African front. Her fashion proclivities, however, routinely tested the patience of her superiors. As my mother tells it, an unwillingness to cut her hair to an above-the-shoulder bob cost her a promotion from lieutenant to captain. When my mother passed away, my aunt gave my sister and me letters she had received from my mother during her long tour of duty. Since the mail was censored, large portions of the letters were redacted. However, what remained gave us insight into what our mom went through. Like other soldiers, she requested care packages from home. Rather than asking for her favorite candy bars and shampoo, my mom wanted clothes. No, she didn't want essentials like underwear and socks; instead, she asked for cashmere sweaters and silk blouses! My aunt also received marching orders to buy these items at two of my mother's then favorite stores, Macy's and B. Altman & Co. in New York.

I'll never know if Mom ever received the items, and if she did, whether she wore those fine things. Maybe these clothes reminded her that, in spite of the horrors of war, she was still glamorous Peggy from Queens, New York. Or perhaps she saved them for dates with a certain young soldier from the Army Corps of Engineers whom she married as soon as the two of them returned home safely. Yes, this handsome gentleman was my dad.

A CLOSET FULL OF MEMORIES

The connection that women develop with clothes is undeniable. As Margaret Spencer emphasized in my stylist training course, "One's clothing is as close as one's skin, and is seen as an extension of oneself." The closet edit appointment illustrates this point very clearly. When I conduct a closet edit, some clients are reluctant to part with items because of the associations with them. Reviewing the contents of a closet often resembles a walk down memory lane. There is the dress worn to a child's christening, graduation, or while on a memorable vacation. Clients also hold onto clothes they wore when they were twenty years younger or several sizes smaller.

The DRES System Stylist's training program emphasizes how to go through the wardrobe edit process with empathy and respect. This training includes suggestions about how to frame comments using neutral language to avoid sounding critical. I routinely use *I* statements rather than *you* statements with clients to promote positive interaction known as *dialogue* (*Human Communication: The Basic Course*, Joseph A. DeVito, 2009).

What distinguishes dialogue from conversation is that both individuals listen and speak, and the goal is mutual respect and understanding. In an *I* statement, the speaker expresses a thought or feeling and then offers a reason for the thought. Rather than say, "You look washed out in beige," I would say, "I prefer you in another color that brings out your porcelain complexion." Because *I* statements merely express an explanatory opinion, they run a reduced risk of intimidating a client or making them feel coerced into a decision. Doing our jobs properly requires honesty and the ability to know what to say and how to say it.

We let clients know that we are there to offer a trained point of view, not to tell them how they should dress. If a client really wants to keep an item of clothing that doesn't match her profile, then I follow Tim Gunn's mantra of "Make it work!" This might involve belting a boxy jacket or wearing a cardigan in an optimal color over a blouse in a less pleasing shade.

As a DRES System–Certified Personal Stylist, my ultimate goal is empowerment through style. To encourage style confidence, I ask my clients questions such as the following: "How do you see yourself in this dress?" And "Which top do you prefer?" Or "Tell me the reasons why you like these slacks so much?" To reinforce the learning process, I also regularly ask clients to clarify what they have learned about how to dress for their body type or style personality. "So what makes this an ideal dress for your body type?"

STYLE RUNS DEEP

An amalgamation of factors such as race, ethnicity, religion, economic status, and family background all play a pivotal role in shaping one's style attitudes and practices. How one's style develops depends upon the messages they've received from their family, friends, and community as well as the societal mores that prevailed in their developmental years.

My next-door neighbor of twenty years in Washington, D.C., grew up in the San Francisco area. Her name is Anneliese, and she is African American. The influence of her race and sense of belonging to the African American community on her style evolution are undeniable. As a child, Anneliese was taught that her appearance greatly influenced how others perceived her. Consequently, her clothes were always clean and neatly pressed. She even pressed her hair with an iron in lieu of using chemical straightening treatments. Anneliese understood that her behavior in public needed to match her impeccable image.

As Anneliese grew older, she learned more clearly how image could be used to shape perceptions. She watched her mother go to great lengths each morning to apply her makeup and put on custom-made suits and matching hats to go to work. Anneliese received a great deal of her style education from her grandmother, who taught her the value of choosing quality over quantity. The white families who employed Anneliese's grandmother routinely gave her gently used clothing from the city's finest department stores like I. Magnin & Co. and Gump's. To this day, a woolen blue and gray houndstooth jacket with custom buttons from her grandmother hangs in Anneliese's closet.

Anneliese believes that the emphasis that African Americans place on image stems partly from a desire to reverse negative stereotypes and shape new, positive perceptions. Writers have also theorized that the tendency of African Americans to dress elegantly is connected with their history of being denied an opportunity to acquire status in other ways (*The Language of Clothes*, Alison Lurie, 1981).

As Anneliese recalls, the turmoil of the 1960s empowered blacks to redefine themselves by embracing their African roots. Many chose to display their cultural pride by wearing natural hair styles and African-inspired clothing, like dashikis. This time for Anneliese was marked by self-discovery. On "free dress" day, while a student at the Katherine Delmar Burke School for Girls in San Francisco, Anneliese wore bell-bottoms instead of her school uniform and styled her hair in an Afro. As she walked her usual route from the bus stop through the exclusive Pacific Heights neighborhood to her school, the police followed her the entire time. At the age of only fifteen, she learned that there were consequences associated with self-expression through style, especially for a person of color.

The influences in Anneliese's life left an indelible mark on her style identity and habits. Good grooming still forms the foundation of her image, and she regularly invests money on personal grooming services. I rarely see Anneliese without a striking new coiffure, and a fresh manicure and pedicure. Anneliese's style personality also reflects her early introduction to well-tailored clothing as well as her creative and adventurous spirit. She looks equally at home in designer jeans and a simple leather jacket or a Moroccan print caftan and chandelier earrings.

My neighbor in Greenville, Lola, is first-generation Mexican American and spent her entire life in Greenville. I can always count on lovely Lola to model the latest fashion trends, which she wears so well. Every year she and her family return to her parents' village in Mexico for visits. Like Anneliese's family, Lola's mother also taught her ten children lessons about image through her example.

Even when Lola's mom went to the grocery store, she dressed meticulously from head to toe. Lola's family also believed in dressing up in their finest clothes for church and family gatherings. Lola traces this custom to the Mexican cultural tradition of congregating at *la plaza* in the evenings to walk, socialize, and dine. Lola's non-Latino friends noticed and often commented on the fact that other Latinos in Greenville wore what they described as "prom dresses" to the mall. Before the revitalization of downtown Greenville, the mall was the closest facsimile to *la plaza* that existed in the city.

Religious beliefs and experiences with religious institutions also influence the development of attitudes about style and style expression. I was raised Catholic, came from a culturally Catholic family, and also attended parochial schools through the eleventh grade. Although many of the nuns who educated me back in the 1950s and 1960s were nurturing teachers, the church had its share of individuals who received their training at "Attila the Hun" University. Often these individuals assumed the role of style enforcers and, on more than one occasion, singled me out for my crimes of fashion. The church enforced a litany of unwritten rules back then, and the majority of them targeted girls. To keep our Eve-like seductive powers in check, black patent leather shoes, which apparently reflected up one's dress, and skirts that bared the knees were strictly taboo. During gymnasium dances, the nuns at my school tapped girls (and not boys) on the shoulder during slow dances to remind them to make room for the Holy Ghost.

I remember one incident very clearly even after fifty years. The year was 1959. That year my elementary school instituted air raid drills, which consisted of marching single file out into the hallway and sitting on the floor with our backs against the wall. How this practice would save us from nuclear annihilation remains a mystery to me to this day.

One day that year, I got dressed in a baby-blue, classic crew-necked, pullover sweater and a navy pleated skirt. My mom fixed my hair in a ponytail and wound a matching ribbon around it. Off I went to school feeling really good about myself. The feeling was short-lived. When Sister Saint Anthony saw me sitting in my fifth grade homeroom, she gave me the evil eye and ordered me into the hall. There she accused me of dressing like "a hussy" and forbade me from wearing another tight-fitting sweater to school ever again. Apparently, she deemed my ponytail too risqué for a ten-year-old, and ordered me to take it down on the spot.

When my mother picked me up from school that fateful day, the first words out of my mouth were "What's a hussy?" My mother immediately transformed into an Irish Ninja and went in search of Sister Saint Anthony. When she returned to the car, she said nothing about her conversation with my teacher. The next day she styled my hair in the same ponytail and told me that I need not worry about anything. She was right.

Hats off to all those moms in the world, like mine, who rescue their children from the tyranny of others. Thanks to my mom, my budding style gene remained undamaged. I tested the good sisters on a number of occasions after that. I even dared wear a sleeveless dress to my eighth-grade graduation and almost got yanked out of the procession to receive my diploma.

People throughout the world publicly pronounce their religious beliefs and affiliations through their clothing. I interviewed a young woman named

Tehseen for this chapter. Tehseen currently lives in Washington, D.C., and clerks for a federal judge. Her family came from India, but she was born and raised in the suburbs of Chicago. Raised as a Muslim, she practices the religion of Islam. Tehseen identifies herself as Muslim, American, and South Asian. Her faith requires her to cover every part of her body except her face, hands, and feet and to wear a *hijab*, or head scarf.

Tehseen pays attention to her image. She wants to represent herself and her faith well, and also dress in accordance with her personality and style preferences. Her South Asian heritage and her contemporary tastes show up in the lively patterns, rich textures, and colors she wears. She loves flowing chiffons, and shiny silks in mauve and sea mist with intricate beaded or sequin work. As her professional career evolves, Tehseen enjoys creating work-appropriate and strikingly elegant outfits that match her personal style.

While in elementary school, Tehseen experienced her share of taunting for wearing customary South Asian–style pants with her dresses. Once she entered high school, the teasing stopped. She attributes this behavior shift to her classmates' increased maturity. A quiet and studious young woman, Tehseen also began wearing the *hijab* at that time. Her nunlike appearance might have also encouraged her classmates' deference.

STYLE GEOGRAPHY

Having lived all over the United States and in England while growing up, I tune into how geography impacts style. As a recent transplant from Washington, D.C., to Greenville, South Carolina, I'm also learning more about the style differences between these two cities. I laugh every time I read Tim Gunn's description of D.C. as a "fashion desert" (*Tim Gunn: A Guide to Quality, Taste and Style,* Tim Gunn with Kate Moloney, 2007).

The thirty-six years that I spent in D.C. gave me plenty of time to ponder why Washington has developed a reputation for not being the nation's fashion capital. I use three *S* words to describe D.C.'s style: serious, sedate, and sensible. So many D.C. area dwellers rely on a uniform of sorts to suit their work-driven, seventy-hour workweek lifestyle. The basic power suit with minimal accoutrements simplifies dressing and fits the bill for function and appropriateness. I also believe this style uniformity levels the playing field. No one has to expend any energy interpreting the nuances of another's clothing, nor do they get easily distracted by them.

I think Tim Gunn would be pleased by the recent styling up of his hometown. Young people and people from all over the globe flock to D.C. and leave their fashion imprint. As neighborhoods evolve, their style follows suit. A walk down K Street provides a much different visual experience than a stroll along U Street. On K Street, black, gray, and navy suits abound while U Street has its share of skinny jeans in living color and fashion-forward fedoras. How grateful I am for this much needed dose of color!

In her book *The Language of Clothes*, Alison Lurie identified the Deep South as a regional style. I can't comment on whether Greenville's style represents that deep southern regional style, but I do see definite style differences between Greenville and D.C. women: Greenville women look more done up. Their hair looks more intentionally styled. They wear more color, more jewelry, more hats, more dresses, and less practical, prettier shoes. Living here has rubbed off on me. I've gone blonder, and my hair is more layered. For the first time in my life, I go to a salon just to get my hair washed and styled. I also now follow a multistep skin care regimen that involves applying a drawer full of Mary Kay products to my face and hands daily. Oh, and I also wear higher heels now, especially with my slim-cropped slacks.

New York and Paris are two of the best cities for people watching on this planet. In Paris, women of all ages look chic beyond belief. Just how do they make sartorial magic out of a few simple items of clothing?
Fashion 101 must be a prerequisite in all French schools. My elegant, fifty-something friend Kit travels to Paris often. Like the French, she can milk the

heck out of a scarf or a statement necklace. From time to time we muse about what constitutes the essence of French glamour.

According to Kit, it all boils down to quality, simplicity, and age appropriateness. In other words, the French live by two fashion tenants: "Less is more" and "Quality over quantity." Mature French women also don't feel the need to dress or look like teenagers. However, they take care of themselves and don't spiral down to frumpiness. French men also fawn over any elegant woman, regardless of her age. Kit recently enjoyed the respectful attention of a waiter at a Paris bistro who had an eye for sophistication. Elegance, and not age, matters to the French. What a refreshing concept.

Attitude is everything in New York City. New Yorkers have the swagger to pull off just about any imaginable fashion concoction. On a trip there one summer, my husband and I headed to the famous Blue Note Café in the West Village to listen to some jazz. As we stepped out of the cab, a couple strolled by arm in arm down the street. The woman wore a full-length sheer white slip, as distinguished from a slip dress, bikini underwear, and flip-flops. What amazed me more than her over-the-top outfit was the fact that no one seemed even remotely phased by it. If one feels like breaking free of their style inhibitions, I recommend, for inspiration's sake, visiting the city where anything goes.

STYLE MATTERS

Whether one lives in New York or Nebraska, style matters. All of us rely on what we see to form impressions of others. Studies show that erasing a bad first impression takes some doing. Image, a critical data point in all relationships, includes appearance, social skills, and body language.

When searching for a possible mate, we take into consideration a person's grooming, their physical features, and their clothing. We hone in on the qualities that attract a person to us. Perhaps an athletic build in a man speaks to us, or maybe we notice a man in an exquisitely tailored suit. We receive visual cues and interpret them based on our intuition and our storehouse of experiences. We then use that information to navigate the relationship waters. This is how we conclude that someone has kind eyes, a welcoming smile, or a confident walk.

No one can refute the significance of image in the work world. Most companies establish written dress policies to encourage their employees to represent them well. Employers pay close attention to appearance and draw conclusions about an employee's performance based on this factor. A well-dressed employee often appears more organized than a less attractively attired coworker. Being properly dressed may also signify a level of involvement that favorably impresses employers (*The Language of Clothes*, Alison Lurie, 1981).

A phenomenon called the "halo effect" applies here. Individuals who view others' appearance in a positive light automatically attribute a host of additional positive characteristics to that person (www.experiment-resources.com/halo-effect.html). As an example, attractive people are seen as better networkers, and are thought to be more persuasive and principled than less attractive individuals (www.askmen.com/feeder/askmenRSS_article_print_2006.php?ID=1045529).

The benefits of being attractive also affect the size of one's paycheck. According to the results of a 2009 study, attractiveness is linked to higher incomes and less financial strain (*Journal of Applied Psychology* 94, no. 3, Timothy A. Judge, Charlice Hurst, Lauren S. Simon, 2009).

As an explanation, the study cites the fact that attractive people believe in their own self-worth and capabilities. Interestingly enough, one's perceived attractiveness and intelligence had a larger effect than attractiveness, and as strong an effect as intelligence on income. This conclusion illustrates the self-fulfilling-prophecy concept at work. Positive beliefs fuel self-confidence. Self-confidence encourages positive behaviors. Positive behaviors shape reality.

JOB INTERVIEW: WHERE THE STYLE STAKES ARE HIGH

Job interviews provide individuals with a very narrow window in which to wow prospective employers. It goes without saying that employers and recruiters scrutinize each candidate's image and weigh that along with other key factors. In an article that I wrote for the Greenville, South Carolina, edition of Examiner.com titled "How to Dress for a Job Interview," I interviewed members of Greenville's business community on the subject of appropriate interview attire. Everyone I interviewed rated the importance of an interviewee's overall image as 10 (extremely important) on a scale of 1 to 10. The community manager of a large apartment complex in Greenville shared her impressions of candidates who fail to dress for success. "If they do not care about the way they look, why should they care about their performance at work?" (www.examiner.com/fashion-trends-in-greenville/how-to-dress-for-a-job-interview).

Apparently other employers share this sentiment. Over 150 employers nationwide cited negative image as the top reason why job candidates were eliminated from consideration after a first interview.

I devised an easy, winning interview image formula that I call B.E.S.T. Following this basic, elegant, simple, and tasteful approach will result in a polished and appropriate image. Here are a few words about how to look your B.E.S.T. in an interview:

- **B is for Basic:** Stick to neutral-colored suits or dresses that are of the highest quality one can afford.
- **E is for Elegant:** Go for classic core and accent pieces in distinctive fabrics with clean lines. One can always infuse more personal style with tasteful accent pieces.
- **S is for Simple:** "Simplicity is the ultimate sophistication," Leonardo da Vinci wrote. A candidate's performance, rather than their appearance, should take center stage. Too many adornments cause sensory overload and distract others.
- **T is for Tasteful:** Avoid loud prints, strong perfume, oversized or excessive jewelry, and too much makeup. If one's style runs on the

flamboyant side, I suggest repeating the mantra "understated" over and over again while dressing for a job interview.

In a 2006 survey conducted by the National Association of Colleges and Employers, the state of one's grooming made the strongest impact on employers (www.ehow.com/info8311493importance-appearance-job-interview.html). Undoubtedly, grooming plays a key role in image management. If one's hair is unkempt, clothes rumpled, or shoes not shined, not even an Armani suit can redeem these image faux pas. In today's job market, marshal every available resource to get a foot in the employer's door. A positive appearance can give just the needed edge over another, less well-groomed candidate with equal qualifications.

SUITED FOR EXCELLENCE

A recent study from the Kellogg School of Management at Northwestern University found that dress affected how test subjects performed. The subjects who wore white lab coats made about half as many errors on a test as their non-lab-coat-attired peers. The subjects who were told that their white coats were artists' smocks did not score above average on their performance test. The study suggests that the wearing of certain clothes, coupled with the meaning that individuals assigned to them, affects performance ("What You Wear Could Affect How Well You Work," Jena McGregor, *Washington Post,* March 2012).

Those who want to function at the top of their game may get a considerable boost by dressing in clothes they associate with power and confidence. If additional research supports the Kellogg School's findings, then individuals and corporations might make these modifications:

- Telecommuters will change out of their bathrobes and into work casual attire before sitting at their computers each day.

- Corporations might rethink the wisdom of their casual Friday dress policies.
- Individuals will give more thought to how they feel in certain types of clothes.

Some already think that relaxed dress codes are leading us down a slippery slope to sloppy. Here is one writer's take on casual day: "Casual Friday soon turned into laissez-faire Monday, takin'-out-the-trash Tuesday, sweatpants Wednesday, and 'Dude!' Thursday" (*I Love You—Now Hush*, Melinda Rainey Thompson and Morgan Murphy, 2010).

For business owners and entrepreneurs, personal image and business brand go hand in hand. Growing a successful business today requires a well-designed website and a strategic online marketing strategy. One's brand should convey a consistent and powerful message. These methods alone won't guarantee customers, however. In the end, the secret to success involves old-school relationship building. Those who engage in face-to-face networking and present a purposeful image will get noticed. They will also get customers. Business owners market themselves wherever they go and with every waking hour of every day. In other words, it pays to always look good and act well.

LIFE LESSONS

Every situation in life provides an opportunity to further professional and personal goals. Anyone could meet their future spouse, close friend, or next big client at the grocery store. Underestimating the power of image never pays off. You step into the limelight every time you walk out your door. Wearing pajama bottoms and stretched-out sweats as casual wear exemplifies poor image management. I am in no way suggesting that appearance is everything. No one achieves success in life by merely looking good. Those who possess form but no substance advance just so far in life before their personal deficiencies become apparent.

Individuals who succeed do so because they believe in excellence. There is no substitute for drive, preparation, and education. Time must be invested in being the best in every area, including appearance.

"Strong lives are motivated by dynamic purposes."
—Kenneth Hildebrand

COLOR COMPLEXITIES

I thank the DRES System Color Analysis training for opening my eyes to the transformative power of color. A recently renewed interest in color by designers and retailers has trickled down to consumers. More women are bravely wearing neon green, cobalt blue, and hot pink.

Color can either be a friend or foe. I've seen some examples of color blocking gone wild that literally cause eye strain. On the other hand, something magical happens when individuals use color correctly. One of my clients stands close to six feet tall and has an imposing frame. It is difficult to fail to notice her. Nevertheless, when she wears certain colors, she begins to recede into the background. Her legs don't seem quite as long; her large expressive eyes get overlooked. After analyzing her color, I determined that she scored a home run with colors like teal, ruby, and green-gray. Both my client and I also observed that a bronze-gold made her complexion glow.

When she tried on a long-sleeved, draped-neck teal top and a metallic python print shell underneath a beige-gold sweater shrug, we both stared at the mirror with our mouths agape. Neither one of us could ever have imagined how drop-dead gorgeous she looked. All of her best assets suddenly ratcheted up a notch.

Well-known stylists Jesse Garza and Joe Lupo discuss the emotions that color produces in individuals in their book *Life in Color: Visual*

Therapy's Guide to the Perfect Palette—for Fashion, Beauty, and You! Colors impact mood and behavior. They alter certain physiological responses such as heart rate, respiration, and blood pressure. Studies show that the color red increases respiration while blue slows it down.

Garza and Lupo point out that orange and yellow stimulate appetite. Pink lowers aggression, and purple emanates spirituality. Greens are associated with harmony and balance, while navy blue is a cerebral shade. That ubiquitous red power suit connotes assertiveness and charisma, and red increases eye-blink frequency whereas blue decreases it (*Human Communication, the Basic Course*, Joseph A. DeVito, 2009).

So should one select a color based on the emotions that it generates? Wearing colors purely for their emotional impact often creates the opposite effect than the one desired. Color-savvy individuals know how to convey an emotion using an accent color. A red and gray print top, paired with a gray suit in lieu of a solid red suit, sufficiently powers a look without going overboard. Politicians on the campaign trail use this technique when they wear red ties with their blue suits.

People should select color based on their complexion, hair, and eyes, and body type. A Sapphire should wear darker colors on the bottom and lighter ones on the top, while a Ruby should do just the opposite. In the inimitable words of Coco Chanel, "The best color in the world is the one that looks good on you."

That is why the DRES System Color Analysis is such a critical styling service. I advise everyone to discover their forty-two Ultimate Colors using the DRES System's color analysis method. Whenever I go shopping, I take my personalized DRES System forty-two Ultimate Colors Palette insert with me to ensure that I've selected just the right shade of blue or green for my hair, eyes, and skin.

Knowing which colors to wear and when to wear them requires good judgment and skill. Never wear red to a job interview; stay with neutrals and wear select colorful accent pieces. Color experts advise that defense attorneys wear blue rather than black or brown to inspire trust and confidence. "Black is so powerful, it could work against the lawyer with the jury. Brown lacks sufficient authority" (*Human Communication, the Basic Course*, Joseph A. DeVito, 2009).

ALL WOMEN ARE GEMS

When I discovered the DRES System, I knew I'd found an organization that spoke my language. From the start, the DRES System's mission to improve the way people view their bodies impressed me. I found the method of body-type classification using precious gemstones a welcome departure from the unflattering fruit labels. I enjoy telling women that they are shaped like a gemstone because this positive association alone reinforces the belief that everyone radiates beauty.

This quote by Sophia Loren epitomizes the DRES System's philosophy: "Feeling good about oneself is the connection between beauty and self-image. The more comfortable you are in your own skin, the more beautiful you are."

Margaret Spencer created the DRES System with this purpose in mind: to help women shed their negative self-perceptions and embrace their body shapes. This thread runs through every step of the styling process.

A poor body image corrodes self-image. In the opinion of body image expert Dr. Thomas F. Cash, the relationship we have with our bodies influences as much as one-third of our overall self-esteem. In a 2004 study dealing with body image among college students, 46 percent of participants displayed difficulties or dissatisfaction with their body image. In half of that group, the seriousness of the difficulties hampered daily living. A negative body image can lead to depression, eating disorders, and a condition called body dysmorphic disorder, a completely distorted body concept (*The Body Image Workbook: An Eight-Step Program for Learning to Like Your Looks*, Thomas F. Cash, 2008).

Inspired by my DRES style training, I came up with an idea to boost the self-image of clients and those who follow my blog. I became familiar with the effectiveness of affirmations during my work in the counseling field, and also liked the fact that the DRES System asks clients to write their style statement as an affirmation.

Why not write style affirmations? I began posting them regularly on both my blog and the DRES System's blog. My themes vary from improved posture to making peace with bathing suits. They usually follow a set formula. I first state the affirmation and then follow it with an explanation of its value. I end with suggestions for practice. Here is one that I share with clients before we embark on a shopping trip together: "I am a mindful shopper. Shopping requires a positive attitude, time, and patience."

Rushing out at the last minute and hurrying to buy something is almost always a recipe for disaster. Another common shopping pitfall is expecting that you will find what you are looking for right away. Mindfulness is as essential to shopping as it is to any of life's tasks. By slowing down, removing expectations, and staying in the moment, you will be far more likely to find what you want without the stress and fatigue often associated with this process. I ask my clients to repeat this affirmation before and during each shopping outing. I also ask for feedback on how this practice works for them.

Affirmations help us bring about what we desire by repeating statements that keep our thoughts in the present. Affirmations encourage us, limit undue negative thinking, and promote positive action. Our minds constantly process information and engage in inner monologue to help us interpret everything we experience.

Psychotherapist Albert Ellis labeled this dialogue "self-talk." He popularized the revolutionary but simple theory that thoughts cause feelings. According to Ellis, thoughts in and of themselves are neutral. It is one's interpretation of a thought that causes a feeling. According to Ellis, individuals need not be slaves to their negative emotions. They can change their feelings by changing their learned thought patterns (*Thoughts & Feelings: Taking Control of Your Moods & Your Life*, Matthew McKay, Martha Davis, Patrick Fanning, 2011).

Affirmations are one proven way to reverse self-sabotaging thought patterns that cause negative emotions. To be effective, they should be short and framed in the present, as if the desired outcome is achieved (www.vitalaffirmations.com/affirmations.htm). Let's say an individual just got promoted to an executive assistant position, which requires good time management and organization skills. This individual feels anxious about being able to handle the additional responsibilities of the job. A suitable affirmation for this situation might be "I am efficient and excel at multitasking."

The Women's Institute for Financial Education (WIFE) is a nonprofit organization to help women gain financial independence. This organization included a *money-attraction affirmation* in one of their recent monthly newsletters (www.wife.org). It beautifully sums up the purpose and power of affirmations: "If you believe it, you can achieve it."

DRES Stylists are change agents. We help change the meanings attached to thoughts, behaviors, and lives through the vehicle of style, one individual at a time. We celebrate each time an individual lets go of their limiting beliefs and fears and discovers their full potential. Leading a complete life means daring to step into the spotlight and embracing all of life's possibilities. Martina Navratilova encourages others to lead dynamic and boundless lives. "I think the key is for women not to set any limits." Are you ready to live your best life?

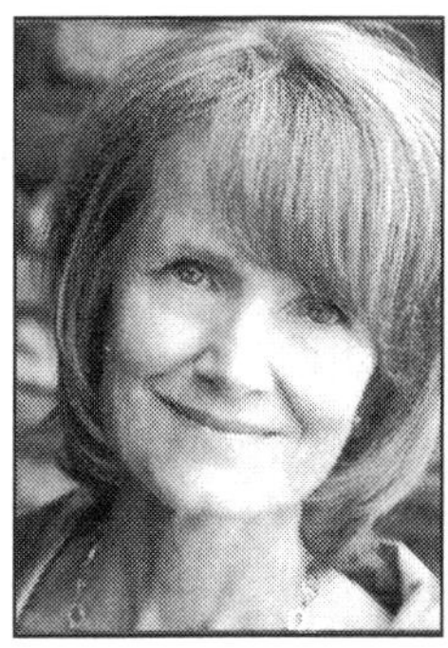

Corey Urbina

DRES System–Certified Personal Stylist

Style Matters
www.stylemattersgreenville.com
corey@stylemattersgreenville.com
Greenville, South Carolina

Two words best describe Corey Urbina's professional life—diverse and multidimensional. She holds an A.B. degree in English and a Masters in Counseling. Before discovering wardrobe styling, Corey spent fifteen years in both fitness and social work.

As a fitness specialist, Corey comanaged an exercise studio in Washington, D.C., where she taught aerobics, trained instructors, and conducted wellness programs. In 1986, she started Body Business, a personal training and corporate fitness company.

In her next career, Corey managed nonprofit and government social service programs. She served as assistant director of a sexual assault center, a youth education advocate, and parent education coordinator for Arlington County, Virginia.

In 2006, Corey began volunteering at two nonprofit organizations for women seeking employment. There she helped individuals select professional attire and conducted career development seminars. Corey not only derived satisfaction from her work, but she also realized her wardrobe styling talent.

Corey's volunteer experience motivated her to pursue additional style training. She worked in retail sales at Nordstrom and at a Washington, D.C., boutique. Corey completed the DRES System stylist training program, and also became certified in color analysis and men's styling.

Corey jokes that she saved her third and best career for last. In 2010, Corey started her own wardrobe styling business, Style Matters, and two years later moved it from D.C. to Greenville, South Carolina.

CHAPTER 3

TRENDS

YOU DONT NEED THEM ALL

By Kira Brown

"I just spent $350 at the mall on what's in style right now, and I still have nothing to wear!"

Have you ever said this to yourself? I often found these words coming out of my mouth each and every time I went shopping. That was before I discovered the DRES System and how trends can work for or against my best personal style. And I have heard a similar complaint about spending money and still not having anything to wear time and time again with my clients. Complaints like "I bought a black tank top, a pastel floral top, one pair of pink skinny jeans, one pair of dark purple harem pants, two pairs of boot-cut flared denim jeans. All because that's what was on the racks and what the magazines tell me is in style, and I still have nothing to wear!" All these trends and nothing to wear! So where are trends going wrong for us and how can we make them right for us? Let's explore trends in depth and discover the value of trends in your DRES System wardrobe.

Trends are essential for keeping your image and your core wardrobe investment current. A core wardrobe is a base collection of foundation pieces that reflect your best personal style, which you can build on to make a complete wardrobe. Chosen trends in clothing, accessories, jewelry, makeup, and even hairstyles can easily update your DRES System core wardrobe collection, adding a fresh and modern twist of style to your basics that help you transition from season to season, day to night or just transform a tired outfit with less cost than a fresh new seasonal wardrobe. Trends can also add a variety of styles to layer onto your own best style.

Often my clients will run to the stores to buy the latest collection or pieces and have no strategy for the trend or how it fits into their current stage of life, wardrobe goals, and overall image goals. With the variety and agility of quickly changing trends from designer to designer, from season to season, how does the mania of trends fit into the DRES System of a balanced wardrobe and life?

Beginning with what I describe as the truth about trends and ending with what trends warrant a "trend spend," let's explore the fashion phenomena and when trends fit best into a balanced wardrobe to keep you best dressed for you, your body, and your best personal style.

THE TRUTH ABOUT TRENDS

If you're trendy or wearing something that's on trend, what does that really mean? With the consumer influence of trendy stores like H&M or Zara, trends have become a way of fashion life. Perhaps we either overlook or overemphasize trends when analyzing a complete wardrobe and efficient shopping strategy to enhance one's style and wardrobe image.

I consider trends to be a certain style that is most popular for its market (fashion, jewelry, accessories, and so on during a particular time period or season). In sum, being on trend is when you are in with the current fashion, as opposed to when, as Heidi Klum from *Project Runway* is famous for stating, "One minute you can be in and the next, you're out." In fashion, trends differ from classic, timeless pieces of clothing, accessories, and jewelry found in a wardrobe that has sustained time and trend cycles. Depending on the piece, classics are styles of certain clothing that fit easily into any season of style, no matter the current trend. On the other hand, trends are perceived to be wearable only for a certain period or time, such as a three-month season.

I love trends. They're fun, and they keep the flow of fashion moving, but trends can become overwhelming without knowledge and a plan! Trends that used to change seasonally can now change monthly. I love giving tips on why trends are important in our dress and how to effectively incorporate them into your best personal style with ease.

In fashion and beauty, trends are big business worldwide. The global economy of fashion is seemingly obsessed with ever-changing trends, with countless magazines and major media outlets, blogs, Twitter feeds, and more updating information daily about new trends. And with the popularity of our celebrity-centric pop culture in recent years, trends have become even more of a hot topic as we Americans devour the trends of our favorite celebrities. From Jennifer Lopez for Kohl's to Gwenyth Paltrow for Tod's to Sarah Jessica Parker for Halston Heritage, celebrities are a major catalyst to what's in for the season or just the moment.

DEFINING TRENDS

When researching the definition of trends, a certain reference caught my eye on dictionary.com, the definition of trends: "The general course or prevailing tendency; drift." That's certainly the case with trends. Trends are the general course of any given season, most often categorized as fall/winter and spring/summer. Some fashion houses even further categorize trends with subsets of wearable times such as resort wear or *prêt-à-porter* (ready to wear) or most recently, "pre-fall" or "pre-summer." With these types of trend categorizations, it's easy to notice that trends are designed to rotate and expire within a one-year time span at most.

Though by definition trends are a prevailing tendency, with the vast number of designers, manufacturers, and other influencers of trends, trends can vary from company to company, from fashion business to fashion business, from market to market under the umbrella of the multibillion-dollar fashion and beauty industry with little or no correlation from one trend to the next . The variety and combination of trends is seemingly endless. During a selected season, the prevailing trend among fashionistas could be as subtle as the most popular color of the moment woven into many styles at Anthropologie, to a more dramatic style of fashion such as brightly colored tunics and patterned stockings found at Tory Burch. Similarly, in accessories trends, one season the trend could be ladylike jewelry from Tiffany & Co. to a completely different, even opposing trend of rocker chic from Kara Ross. With this, choosing the right trend for you each season can be overwhelming without the guidance of your personal DRES System Stylist.

WHERE DO TRENDS COME FROM?

Trends can be described as the creative and continuous flow of the fashion and beauty industry, dictated by many factors. First, international haute couture fashion houses and acclaimed upscale designers such as Chanel, Louis Vuitton, Prada, Michael Kors, Kate Spade, Tory Burch, and others define trends for their brands each season, with each collection from their own inspirations and ideas. The seasonal ideas of these and other large and influential fashion designers trickle down through the fashion pipeline to the lowest retailers on the totem pole to copy and emulate for their customers. Fashion designers are endlessly quoted in magazine articles and elsewhere on "where their inspiration for each trend comes from."

Couturiers' trends are the most valuable and most expensive due to their originality of design and high quality. When you see a Michael Kors Collection dress priced at $1,500 versus an Michael Kors Lifestyle dress that is similar yet a mere fraction of the cost at $125, be advised that you are paying the higher collection price for the originality of the initial design and the quality of craftsmanship. With runway and collection designs, better fabrics, materials, adornments, and skilled dressmakers are used to execute the idea. And trends bred from exclusive brands tend to generate a limited amount of pieces for each trend, driving the demand up for the newest, most unique, and highest-quality piece of fashion.

- Runway trends can be so outlandish that they fail to trickle down into a larger mass-market store. Some examples of trends that just weren't worth spending on include:
- The Pac-Man Helmet by Giles Deacon for London Fashion Week, 2008—Literally, a helmet that looked like Pac-Man!
- Gareth Pugh's Wizard of Oz collection for London Fashion Week, 2008—Imagine Dorothy.
- Alexander McQueen's ten-inch stiletto boots, though Lady Gaga was seen wearing them in 2011. Not many of us can pull off a Gaga look!
- Adriani Bertini Condom Dresses—yes, colorful and artful dresses made out of condoms. You probably aren't sorry you missed this one either!

Large trends, however, that gain popularity among the shopping masses in a particular market or even worldwide do have the potential for longevity and changeability from one season to the next. We have seen that, for example, in fall/winter 2011, the 1990s made a comeback with large floral prints for jeans. The trend continued into spring 2012 with similar floral prints for shorts and spring dresses. Though most trends will fade, a small percentage of trends will become iconic or classic pieces of fashion and design; for example, flapper-fringe styles. Later in this chapter we will explore some trends that have withstood the test of time.

Trends in fashion originate from an array of inspirations each season and vary from designer to designer. From pop culture to mass media, to nature, other design industries and more, trends in fashion can originate from virtually anywhere. Coco Chanel is famous for saying, "Fashion is not something that exists in dresses only. Fashion is in the sky, in the street; fashion has to do with ideas, the way we live, what is happening."

Large haute couture fashion houses greatly influence the trend market. What you may see on the runway of Versace or Marc Jacobs may have a trickle-down effect to the smallest design retailers as noted before. Their inspiration, however, may have come from a creative epiphany, their lifestyle, or another form of inspiration such as fabrics, for example. Few designers create their own fabrics for design and dressmaking. Fabric makers may introduce a certain shade of orange or a unique pattern into their collections at the industrial level of fashion design, which will in turn influence even the most reputable and most influential fashion houses. And what could have influenced the fabric designer and fashion designer or both could have been something in nature, which is a common influencer among designers, a pop culture trend, a mass media trend, or even a home design trend. In short, the reintroduction of a classic with a fresh, modern twist. These are a few of the most common inspirations for trends and design.

Here are a few quotes from major fashion houses on their inspiration for trends and ideas:

"If you spend your time waiting for the inspiration to come to you, for the ideas to 'gush forth,' it will be too late. It is like with a magazine: there is a deadline . . . we have deadlines and that is a healthy form of discipline. It creates ideas."
—Karl Lagerfeld

"Lots of shine for evening . . . lots of ornamentation with a lot of Art Deco sort-of-feeling to it because, again, I think this collection really is New York. So automatically to me, it's the Chrysler Building."
—Michael Kors

"It's about Old Hollywood glamour, but in a ripped T-shirt kind of way."
—Rick Owens

"It's different things—my house, travel, art. And then what I've been doing for fun lately, which is the little surprise in the show."
—Cynthia Rowley

POP CULTURE AND TRENDS

First, pop culture waves have a huge impact on design and trends. The popular culture of the 1970s or '80s influenced trends in music, fashion, jewelry, home and design, and more. For example, the 1970s' underlying theme of free love, freedom, spirituality, and rebellion against authority launched the colorful, free-flowing aspects of fashion, jewelry, and design. Tie-dye, headbands, piercings, and other trends were to rebel symbolically against the constraints of authority and war.

Similarly, the 1980s' trends of rock metal, hair bands, and underground drug culture influenced designers, musicians, celebrities, and other notables to show a darker time with trends of leather, lace, and loads of makeup and jewelry. The 1980s is also where we started to see many more celebrities, rather than nameless models' faces, endorsing products and appearing on magazine covers. Even this subtrend in fashion and beauty has launched a revolution in the sale of fashion-related products. It's nearly impossible to see an advertisement for a national or international product without a celebrity endorsement, paid or otherwise. This subtrend in fashion and beauty indicates that we trust the opinions of those holding fame and fortune, and that we will sometimes make purchases and investments based on what worked for them without further investigations into products' efficacy, sustainability, background, or more favorable alternatives.

MASS MEDIA AND TRENDS

The mass media have a huge effect on trends as well. Currently, the *Mad Men* cable TV program has spawned a revolution in the 1960s' ladies-in-dresses, men-in-suits trends. This show has become big business in fashion and design, with retailers like Banana Republic focusing their fashion design and their advertising campaigns around *Mad Men* retro style. The trend has spawned not just fashion trends but makeup trends too, with companies including MAC gearing a portion of their advertising dollars and product development toward replicating the *Mad Men* makeup look for women of fresh skin, red lips, and dark, thick eyelashes.

HOME DESIGN AND TRENDS

Home and other design trends, including graphic design and architectural design, can have a direct effect on fashion and beauty trends as well. It's not uncommon to see Martha Stewart Home or Z Gallerie introduce a color palette into their collections and to then begin to see the same or similar palette in fashion and makeup trends. Or, for example, current trends in the past few years for architectural and home interior design trends are focusing on more modern, minimalist design as well as sustainable and eco-friendly design. And this has inspired modern retail designers like Michael Kors to expand his brand into similar boutiques called Lifestyle Stores, which offer modern designs in a similarly modern boutique.

Also, the influx of eco-friendly and organic-sourcing retailers, fabric producers, and designers has skyrocketed in reason years. Eco-friendly products and goods made with sustainable materials and processes can be considered a multidimensional trend encompassing pop culture, design, manufacturing, lifestyles, and even belief systems. Furthermore, eco-consciousness and sustainability may be more than just passing trends, evolving toward a new, modern way of life for the entire world.

THE BIG BUSINESS OF TRENDS

Focusing back to fashion, trends are big business. I was fortunate enough to interview the fashion consultant and mentor, Tim Gunn. I started in fashion as a blogger, founding Fashion Phoenix in 2009. My blog has afforded me amazing opportunities to meet celebrity fashion and style icons. What I loved most about blogging and interviewing are the lessons I learned straight from fashion industry experts like Mr. Gunn. With the following personal gem, he shocked me into changing my personal shopping philosophy and subsequent spending behavior instantly.

He said, "Trends are designed to make buyers run out and spend money." With this, it hit me! I often fall victim to what I call the Trend Spend: spending money on what's new and fresh, just because it's new and fresh, rather than investing smartly in pieces that balance my wardrobe and fill a need in what I have. This vital piece of information about trends and the fashion industry marketplace changed my spending habits for the better, forever. I also realized that trends are big business and influence marketing, sales goals, and consumer behavior.

In my styling practice, I see the Trend Spend time and time again, when men and women buy what's in stores, regardless of whether it is truly "in" for them and their personal style. For example, recently I was asked to style a forty-year-old single mother interested in transitioning her wardrobe from being a married, stay-at-home mother to a working mother ready to enter the dating scene. She bought $350 of trendy new blouses and jeans that didn't fit her age and stage of life. Also, they weren't suited for her body type, which made it difficult for her to find something to wear, though she thought she had bought plenty of options! However, with a careful and honest edit of her new buys, plus a few styling tricks such as layering, we were able to save her $85 in returns for pieces that just wouldn't work and to create multiple outfits that were age-appropriate and current.

The DRES System approaches trends with sensibility and with your personal style and life stage in mind, empowering shoppers to curb unnecessary spending and unnecessary wardrobe volume that can overwhelm your daily ensemble-selection process making it a chore, rather than an exciting start to your day.

THE HISTORY OF TRENDS

As we have touched on previously, trends have played an important role in fashion, especially in the nineteenth century. As opposed to dressmaking, fashion has an important cultural relevance in society. In my interview with Tim Gunn, he stated, "Fashion happens in a context. Dressmaking is just that, making clothing." Fashion is living and ever-changing as society and culture change and evolve. So trends, as an important part of the fabric of the fashion industry at large, change and morph as the industry evolves as well.

As I stated before, some fashion trends will be passing fads, yet some will evolve into classic or even iconic pieces of clothing, and are often symbolic of an era, region, or culture.

Examples of trends across fashion and beauty that have passed like a fad include:

- Bright-blue eye shadow, made popular in the 1970s
- Big hair, perms, and hair teasing of the 1980s
- Acid-washed denim of the 1990s

The list of passing fads and trends that can inspire nostalgia or make you smile and say, "I can't believe I wore that!" could continue at length. What's interesting to note for these passing fads is that often these trends may be reintroduced in the life cycle of the fashion industry in a new way, breathing new life into the trend with a modern take or as a chic, vintage look.

VINTAGE AS TRENDY

Vintage itself has become a modern-day trend. From one perspective, when economic times are tough, as they are today, pulling fashion from the past becomes an economical option to updating one's wardrobe and look. And the term "vintage" itself has such a wide scope of interpretations and definitions that incorporating something vintage into your wardrobe can be both economical and on trend. The exact definition of vintage from the *American Heritage Dictionary* states: "A group or collection of persons or things sharing certain characteristics. . . . A year or period of origin: a car of 1942 vintage."

With these definitions, it's easy to see how pulling your favorite T-shirt from your college years or scoring a great 1980s black cocktail dress from an upscale consignment shop can be perceived as trendy, though neither fit into any certain trend at the moment, other than for the nostalgia and date of origin of the garment.

FROM TREND TO ICON

Although trends are designed to stimulate sales, and then pass on to the next season's trends to again stimulate sales, some trends have become iconic and continue to have influence over the fashion industry and consumer behavior as a whole.

The following are a few of my favorite iconic pieces as mentioned in *Fashion Face-Off: A Trump Card Game* (Maia Adams, Erin Petson: Laurence King Publishing, 2011). *Fashion Face-Off* is a teaching card deck that I use with clients to educate them on trends in a fun way. The following are from my favorite cards that were originally introduced as a trend:

Burberry Trench Coat: Introduced in 1914, the design was originally commissioned for the British War Office during World War I. The coat was created for the soldiers on the front line.

Diane von Furstenberg's Wrap Dress: First introduced in 1972, the DVF wrap dress is a symbol of day-to-day practicality, mixed with the utmost sophistication and style. The wrap dress is still made today and has been rereleased with modern, fresh fabrics to reinvent the classic style again and again. The dress style has also been copied and reinvented by other designers since its inception, more evidence of its influence.

Chanel Suit: The epitome of classic for the contemporary women and fashion lover is the Chanel suit. Coco Chanel herself was one of the most powerful trendsetters of our time with her own personal style of incorporating men's wear into her own daily dress, and the Chanel suit was no exception to her trendsetting power. Traditionally made of tweed and the finest wools, the suit regularly shows up on Chanel runways, though Coco herself died in 1971. Again, Chanel suit styles are replicated by other designers now and still command top dollar for one piece from Chanel. I regularly check high-end fashion consignment shops and eBay waiting to score the perfect jacket to add to my collection at a fraction of the general retail price. A Chanel jacket, with its casual yet sophisticated sense of quality and style, will last in your wardrobe forever. One of my favorite ways it is worn is not as a full suit, but with jeans and high heels, like Cameron Diaz is often seen wearing. It's sophisticated yet age-appropriate for Cameron and for many.

Christian Louboutin Shoes: Christian Louboutin's trendsetting power goes beyond the amazing shoe designs that the fashion designer presents each season. His marketing and branding as the "shoe with the red bottom" started a trend among modern shoemakers to brand their bottoms in color as well. Now the red-soled designer's moniker is considered classic and iconic by fashionistas at large.

The Hervé Léger Bondage Dress: Introduced in 1995, the Herve Leger bondage dress, a tight-fitting dress that molds to the wearer's body, has reached icon status. In its variety of colors and styles, the dress is repeatedly a red carpet pick for svelte-bodied celebrities, even over a decade since its introduction. A Leger replica bondage dress style can routinely be found at the lesser priced, popular sister brand BCBG for a fraction of the cost. As a statement piece, the bondage dress makes quite the, well, statement!

Hermès Birkin Bag: The Birkin bag is the epitome of handbags for die-hard fashionistas. First produced by the French fashion house in 1984, the Birkin was created by Hermès's chief executive, Jean-Louis Dumas, after Jane Birkin, an English actress and singer, spilled the contents of her handbag at the executive's feet during a flight. This little mishap spawned the design of one of the most iconic handbags in history. To keep up with trends, the Birkin bag has been reinvented to add trendy colors and materials to its design. The bag, which retails for roughly $15,000, is more than a trend or an icon; it is a fashion investment. Celebrities are obsessed with their Birkins! I personally love seeing a classic Birkin style in a hot color like lime or hot pink.

The Yves Saint Laurent Tuxedo Suit: During a time when women wore mainly dresses, the YSL tuxedo pantsuit of 1966 was a revolutionary trend in fashion. Symbolic of the women's movement influencing the workplace and of women beginning to break the old norms of "a woman's place is in the home" mentality, the tuxedo pantsuit stormed the fashion scene. Today, the iconic design and cultural norm-shattering fashion trend is reinvented time and time again on the runway and in design. In my opinion, a tuxedo jacket or pants is a wardrobe staple for evening wear. For both men and women, actually! Starting in their thirties, men should have a well-fitting tuxedo for special occasions.

Denim Blue Jeans: Who doesn't love a pair of jeans! Americans live in their denim. What was once considered a uniform for blue-collar workers, wearing denim is now one of the largest revenue sources for fashion. Denim brands try year-round to embody classic cuts and popular trends. And buyers are always particular about their denim and favorite denim styles, as jeans have become a fashion staple for men, women, and children. Denim trends are often reused and reintroduced and are greatly driven by cultural influence. What's more, denim can be trendy, vintage, and classic simultaneously, making for one of the most versatile pieces of fashion available.

The Button-Down Shirt: I love button-downs. They are easy to wear and care for, and come in a wide variety of shades and cuts. Originally designed as a dress shirt for men, a classic white button-down shirt is an iconic piece of fashion for men and women. Brands including Ann Taylor and Ted Baker built their fashion empires on the design and manufacturing of a button-down or similar shirt. Through time, this iconic piece of clothing (not to mention a classic staple piece for any wardrobe) has a unique ability to subtly change and evolve by season with tweaks to the shirt's cuff thickness, length, fabric, and most noticeably, the collar size. Collar sizes and styles for both men and women have important cultural and personal significance. Can you think back to the wide-pointed collars of the 1970s and the *Mary Tyler Moore Show*? And imagine the latest J.Crew catalog filled with button-down shirts with their smaller collars and the bright, bold colors of the season. The button-down shirt has an amazing way to blend its classic style and the most recent trends in fashion. Again, button-downs are a wardrobe staple for men and women.

THE SPEND SPIN

Spending on trends is an important wardrobe tactic for updating your look quickly by purchasing a few key trendy items that complement your wardrobe basics. Spending on trends is also a great way to transition from one season to the next and stay current. Rather than buying an entirely new seasonal wardrobe, a few key trend pieces may function to move from one season to the next with minimal expense and closet storage needs.

Sometimes, though, our trend spending and need to buy, buy, buy something new can initiate what I call the "spend spin." Needless and often unfocused spending on trends, the newest styles, or the latest in stores can conjure up feelings of shopping guilt or worse, a shopping addiction where ever-changing trends can fuel the fire of addictive behavior.

To assess if you fall victim to the spend spin, perhaps take inventory of your closet and spending habits. Do you have clothes with tags still on them? Do you overextend your budget for the latest and greatest trends you see in stores? Is shopping for clothing both a necessary and pleasant experience for you? If you're not sure about these questions or cannot answer them, consult a DRES System Stylist for ways to focus your wardrobe spending appropriately for your lifestyle, body shape, and image goals.

Overall, it is best for most not to splurge until a complete wardrobe assessment has been done. First, editing down to the basic pieces of your wardrobe and then adding complementary trend pieces, is the most sensible way to build a nearly effortless wardrobe.

GETTING PERSONAL WITH TREND SPENDING

Other reasons to avoid overspending get a bit more personal. For example, avoid spending when stressed, sad, or angry. We tend to spend more when we are experiencing unfavorable emotional states than when we are feeling happy. And spending when stressed or sad and, particularly overspending during times of distress, may perpetuate and recycle feelings of guilt and financial stress. Many of us have experienced times when we are shopping our feelings away. The joy of purchasing something new, especially on sale, when emotionally stressed often deflects emotional pain temporarily for some. I know I have tried to buy some happiness from a new dress or new shoes many times. And I have bought many things that I didn't need, and some I couldn't afford, in an attempt to improve my emotional state. Temporarily it worked, but when my credit card bill found its way to my mailbox, the panic and guilt from the shopping spree set in! As mentioned, in extreme cases some turn to shopping addictions to avoid the reality of a larger life problem—many times a larger financial problem.

Other times when trend spending can be problematic are during vacations or between seasons. Vacation spending is often one of the most favorable times to shop. Pre-vacation spending for the perfect outfit to wear, and then more vacation spending for what's in style at the moment, are both popular. However, often we spend and overspend on vacation trends that will last in our wardrobes for mere weeks. Like the time I bought four spaghetti-strap maxi dresses for a trip to Miami. Usually, I don't bare my back or arms when dressing at home but when heading to the beaches of southern Florida, I was inspired to be beachy and show some skin for five whole days with four new dresses! Be careful not to overspend like me on trend wear for short lengths of time. And make sure to spend within your budget.

Trends are the perfect way to transition your base wardrobe from season to season without breaking the bank. Rather than investing in a completely new, seasonal, head-to-toe wardrobe, you can stretch the style longevity of key pieces of fashion, accessories, or beauty trends for weeks, perhaps months.

My personal favorite transitional accessory is the scarf. Scarves in the trendiest colors and fabrics help transition, for example, summer dresses into fall. One of my favorite ways to wear a scarf as a transitional piece is to start with a maxi dress bought during the hot months, topped with a basic jean jacket that's always in my closet, and then affordably updated with a beautiful new scarf tied around my neck in the latest fall color. The cost is minimal, the effort minimal, but the effect on my wardrobe pieces and the satisfaction of having a nearly instant update to my look is tremendous. But beware of spending too much on trends during transitional times, when the weather is changing and sometimes unpredictable. Change can often spur a trend spend spin and a rush to get to the stores for something new to complement the new season.

Finally, spending on last season's trends just because they are on sale can be costly! Sales are those amazing moments when we get something fabulous for a discount. And we love sales, don't we? We all love discounts and deals. Even the wealthiest people love discounts, as reported in the *Business Insider*'s recent article, "Rich People Prefer to Shop at Nordstrom." The article reports that the wealthiest people prefer to shop at Nordstrom versus Barneys New York and Bergdorf Goodman. Nordstrom, opposed to these other two upscale retailers, is known for moderately priced collections, regular discounts, and their half-yearly sales in January and June. Many upscale retailers and design houses have historically opposed discounting their products, until recently, to accommodate the economic downturn. Nevertheless, sales can often be costly when the rush of a great deal trumps the sensibility of a great piece that efficiently balances or complements your wardrobe. I challenge you to shop wisely and sensibly, as do the wealthiest in the world!

WHEN TO AVOID TRENDS

With the wide array of trends, it's important to point out when trends are just wrong for you! There are plenty of times and trends for us all. Avoid trends when they are too young or too old for your lifestyle, when they are not within your budget and, most of all, when they are ultra-gimmicky and over-the-top fads that your gut feeling tells you just won't last. Most likely, you're right!

For example, take the runway shows and garments of the late Alexander McQueen. Many of his garments were pieces of wearable art rather than functional pieces of clothing for everyday wear. The spectacle of the garment construction and overall concept of the designs were often spectacular and trend inspiring, but nonetheless impractical for the masses to wear. Simultaneously, though, an Alexander McQueen dress or garment would be an amazing investment for a special occasion or as a collector's item for the serious fashionista.

A great rule of thumb when buying any trend is if you think it's wrong for you, it is! Trust your gut. Don't waste your time or money, and move on to find what trend pieces make you look and feel like a million bucks. Believe me, with the amount of designers and retailers in the world, the wardrobe pieces that will make you feel amazing are available to you. It just takes some time and patience to find what works best for you; wait for what works the best and don't settle for what "will do." When you do find the perfect complementary trend piece for your wardrobe and fashion goals, most likely the return on your investment on cost per wear and sheer ease of the piece's wearability will be well worth the price and your patience.

Similarly, it is wise to avoid distinct trends for photo-taking opportunities so that a timeless, keepsake photograph can be created. I have had a client, however, who is photographed often as part of his career in the music industry. He told me that each summer during his tour season, he likes to choose a trend for his clothing so that he can differentiate one year from the next. What a great idea! How fun would it be for your family photos to be super trendy year after year and to look back at all the different styles, rather than dressing in classics each year? And that's what I love about fashion in general: it gives you so many opportunities to express yourself.

MEN AND TRENDS

In recent years, men have become an important sector of shoppers for retailers and designers to market to directly. Men's style magazines such as *GQ* and *Details* offer daily tips and trend reports for men exclusively on fashion and grooming practices. It's become trendy for men to focus on trends and what's in style!

I personally find that men who invest in relevant trends for their personal lifestyle, fit, and overall style seem more youthful than others. To explain, the details in the right trends for men (and women) can add to or subtract from the perceived overall fashion sense and style of the wearer. For example, if a forty-year-old man was wearing a tartan plaid shirt with faded, baggy Levi's jeans and Reebok sneakers, he may be perceived as more traditionally manly yet less sophisticated and less trendy than a forty-year-old man in a black blazer and vintage T-shirt, paired with Diesel dark-wash denim jeans and bright blue TOMS shoes. The latter may even be perceived as wealthier than my first example, who is also in baggy jeans. Perceptions in fashion are a large part of being stylish, and trends play an integral part in maintaining or facilitating a stylish perception.

These similar perceptions can hold true for women as well. A lack of trendy pieces can often infer a less-stylish wardrobe and add to the wearer's age, rather than complementing her overall style and embellishing her youthfulness.

DRES FOR TRENDS

In your wardrobe, trends add a touch of time relevance to your style. Adding a variety of styles from a few key trend categories that work for you (or a combination of fashion, beauty, and accessory trends) can freshen up your wardrobe and keep your entire image current, regardless of your personal style, age, or other context. The three main categories of trends I use regularly when updating a client's look are fashion, accessory, and beauty trends. And each trend has many subsets of trends within it, making the accessibility of something fresh viable for anyone on any budget, anywhere.

First, clothing trends vary the most in price, fashion context, and cultural context, and have the most trend subsets from which to choose and integrate into your personal style profile.

In the DRES System, your overall personal style profile is determined by the pre-profile questionnaire, subsequent style assessments, and meetings from which your DRES System Personal Stylist will then help guide you to your best trends. With this, fashion trends can be easily and effortlessly translated into your overall style, making your trend spending deliberate and efficient. And that works best for your wardrobe goals: the right wardrobe trend complementing your main capsule or base wardrobe collection. Within wardrobe trends, the most popular subcategories are fit and color.

TRENDS THAT FIT

Fit

First, let's explore fit trends. Baggy, loose, form-fitting, skinny—fit plays an essential role in wardrobe trends. Depending on the time and context, the fit of the piece can tell you its era. For example, bell-bottom jeans are most likely from the 1960s through '70s; baggy-fit jeans range from the 1980s through '90s.

For the best fitting trends, your DRES System Personal Stylist will take you through the process of finding your personal style; then she'll layer on examples of accessories and trends that complement your best personal style.

Color

Second, is color. Each season there is usually a color change to accompany the change in all designers' collections overall. Colors can change drastically from season to season within one design house to mimic the new collection and to, of course, stimulate sales of the latest and greatest styles. Your personal color selection of your trend pieces can be guided by your DRES System forty-two Ultimate Colors analysis, rather than be dictated by the current season's trend color, depending on your wardrobe needs and goals.

ACCESSORY TRENDS

Accessory trends encompass shoes, jewelry, and adornments of all kinds. Though we have talked about the fashion industry as a whole to include accessory trends, accessory designers can follow their own trend schedule and inspiration independent of garment designers.

Currently, my favorite accessory is shoes. Don't we women love our shoes! Often, just by changing your shoe, you can change the entire look and feel of an ensemble while still being cost-effective. Can you imagine how a simple sheath dress would feel with a pair of black, high-heeled stilettos versus flip-flops? Accessories have the power to change the entire look and feel of an outfit; each season, most design houses infuse their industry with their own seasonal styles.

This is why I love shoes! For transitioning from season to season or just for a special-occasion outfit, shoes make it simple and often less costly than an entire wardrobe overhaul. Recently, my client bought a gorgeous pair of Tory Burch brown leather riding boots. This was the only investment she could make for her new fall wardrobe. Building around just her footwear and the trend of brown, flat riding boots, we mixed and matched day outfits and date-night outfits for her with her existing wardrobe pieces.

We have often heard of many women's shoe collections as being like a library of catalogued brands and styles. Where does this fascination with shoes come from? Perhaps it is a popular trend spend because of the consistency of shoe size. When women avoid shopping because they are ashamed of their bodies or have weight issues, shoes are less intimidating to shop for because weight and perceived body image issues are generally irrelevant to your feet.

Just like shoes, jewelry also has the capacity to change the look and feel of an outfit almost instantly. A basic white tank worn with a small charm pendant necklace has quite a different feel and style to it than the same basic white tank accessorized with ten strands of pearls.

Jewelry recently has become a focus for stand-alone trends and for celebrity endorsements as well. Trends in jewelry can influence designer collections and fashion overall. Trends from bold, layered, and chunky to the simple and understated have come and gone through time. We women love jewelry, and working with the latest jewelry trend can keep your capsule wardrobe current and offer you flexibility to make a statement (or not) with your daily dress.

I like to use a statement piece of jewelry that I wear daily. For me, that is a watch. Though I am a minimalist by nature and prefer to not wear a lot of jewelry, I have to have my watch on! And I like to change my watch styles with current trends. I have chunky watches; dainty watches that my grandmother gave me; smart and small, black leather Audrey Hepburn-inspired watches; and more. My watch is my statement piece, and usually the only piece I consistently wear, besides my stud earrings. But many women, and my clients, love jewelry—layers of jewelry, earrings, and cocktail rings.

What I love about jewelry is that, no matter the trend, quality jewelry can be an almost instant heirloom. I had the privilege to meet Scott Gauthier of Gauthier in Scottsdale, Arizona, an award-winning designer and gemstone collector. While visiting and exploring his extensive collection of rare jewels (some even so rare that the Smithsonian has tried to acquire them!), Gauthier reminded me how an amazing piece of quality jewelry can become an instant family heirloom.

BEAUTY TRENDS

Next, beauty trends can greatly influence your wardrobe and overall sense of fashion. With beauty trends, I love to see how color influences changing styles. For example, a winter look could showcase pale matte skin, dewy red lips, and dark lashes; where a current summer trend could be a pretty pink pout and a dewy, sun-kissed complexion from a sunless tan application and dewy-finish makeup. Beauty, hair, and makeup can be subtle or dramatic, depending on the current trend and how it fits into the context of a woman's life. I always love to wear the latest in nail polish colors to give myself a burst of color and to feel current, for under $10.

Makeup trends are also heavily influenced by runway shows. Haute couture designers don't just design clothing, but integrate hair and makeup looks to complement the vision of their designs, possibly sparking a separate or complementary beauty trend.

YOUR BEST TRENDS

The best trends for you in any category will be based on the results of your DRES System body shape analysis, your DRES face shape analysis, your forty-two Ultimate Colors personal color profile analysis, and your lifestyle. However, the beauty of trends (and not their superficial status as passing fads) is that if you want to dress outside of your style box for that special occasion or big vacation or to fit in with a certain group, the availability, accessibility, affordability, and variety of trends can easily help you achieve that goal.

Trends overall are the perfect complement to update your DRES System–curated wardrobe and overall image. To seasonally transition your wardrobe efficiently and stylishly, strategic trend pieces can be a smart investment for your overall image and in making your daily dressing both easy and enjoyable.

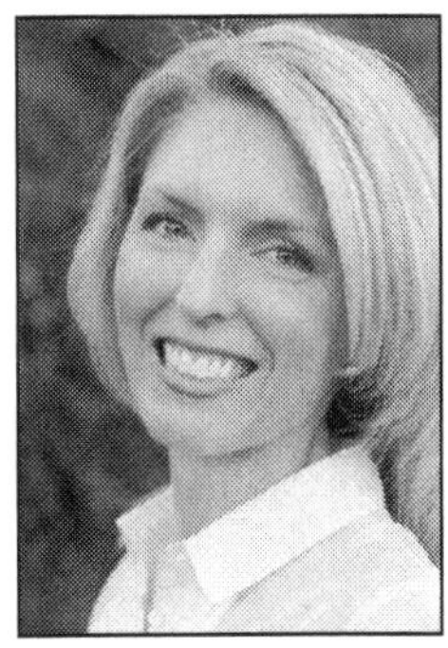

Kira Brown

DRES System–Certified Personal Stylist

Fashion Phoenix

www.fashionphoenix.com

kira@fashionphoenix.com

Phoenix, Arizona

Kira Brown is a communications professional from Phoenix, Arizona. Kira's first move into the fashion industry, beyond regularly swiping her own credit card, was starting the fashion blog FashionPhoenix.com in 2009, where she has interviewed Tim Gunn, celebrity jeweler Neil Lane, Ken Downing of Neiman Marcus, international makeup artist Jemma Kidd, and more.

Kira is a graduate of Arizona State University with a bachelor's degree in human communication, a DRES System–Certified Personal Stylist and a Certified Genius Coach.

In Phoenix, Kira blends her love of fashion, design, and human communication with her background in marketing communications as a marketing and media consultant for fashion and lifestyle brands.

When she's not chatting fashion or marketing, Kira enjoys spending time with her son, practicing yoga, and singing country music.

CHAPTER 4

STYLE

YOUR SIGNATURE LOOK

By Lori Goddard-Weed

Have you ever felt like you grew up in the wrong era for fashion? I was a passionate fan of Doris Day and Jackie Kennedy. Their styles were full of grace and elegance but stayed true to who they were: themselves. I loved the way they were always dressed in classic lines and wore gloves, with handbags and matching shoes. Such ladies, and so very feminine! Their style statements were and still are my passion.

I grew up as something of a tomboy who wanted to wear Levi's jeans, striped T-shirts, and anything that my friends were wearing. Don't get me wrong: I still wanted to be a girly girl, but didn't feel as though I fit that style. Doris and Jackie were grown-ups and I couldn't dress like that. None of my friends were dressing like "old" ladies. I was an athlete: scrappy, rail-thin, lanky, and taller than most of the boys. I was a preteen girl just trying to fit in. But I still loved their style.

No matter what era women live in, they want to look and feel their best; they want to be perceived as beautiful and stylish. I've modeled on and off for years and, being in different shows with different models, I have picked up some new fashion styles, trends, and tips that I subtly tried out. Most models are simply there to work and do the best job they can. However, once in a while I run into another model who seems overconfident and therefore comes across unpleasantly. But for the most part, they are all nice women and we work well together. Sometimes, I work with a model once and then never see her again. Then there are the models whom I've worked with several times and we've built a great rapport. Working well together helps in knowing what to expect from each other, and then we're able to support each other during a show.

In runway modeling, there really is no time to chat between changes. We're all working fast and furiously to make sure to get our next outfit on correctly, and this is when modeling friends and dressers help tuck or tape or pin things to make sure you are looking fabulous and that the garment looks perfect. Socializing with each other is fun but is always left for after the show.

I have received several tips from other models. One of the funniest tips I got involves using panty liners under your armpits, to keep yourself from sweating onto the garment! I had to laugh at this: all I could think of was walking down the runway and having my armpit panty liner slip out, stepping on it, and then finding it stuck to the bottom of my shoe like toilet paper. I would have died of embarrassment with a panty liner stuck on the bottom of my shoe in front of a crowd! Slips, trips, falls, and clothing malfunctions happen but thankfully not very often.

Learning from friends, family, and coworkers is also a great way to make that subtle style change. Try a new look to add a special touch that says *you*. Try out a new way to tie a scarf, braid it for a belt, tie it in your hair in a super chic way, or tie it around a hat to give yourself an ethnic vibe.

Many tips from fashion shows are tricks of the trade to keep our clothing in place with garment tape or to add more curves by putting double pads in bras to model bridal gowns. One of my favorite tips is adding a hairpiece that matches my hair color, giving me a different look during the same show. I can pull up my hair, twist it, add a claw-type clip hairpiece, and voilà! An updo in seconds. And people think it's your own hair pulled up. The look can be very elegant, sassy, or carefree. There are also hair extensions that offer a different look. Your outfit or style choice helps to decide on how to wear your hair. To look a little sassy, your hair should be a little messy, not that smooth nor in a slick -backed bun.

Have you ever tried any type of a body shaper? These are wonderful items to wear to help give the illusion of smoothness. Undergarments are very important. Make sure they fit properly so that your overall look is stunning.

As I entered high school, I wanted to be an awesome athlete, but I also wanted to be a lady. Watching how my mother dressed and entertained was a big influence in my life, as were my high school friends and, later, my college sorority sisters.

My mother worked very hard at her career. For thirty-seven years she worked as a bill dispatcher for a national trucking company. She ran the office, and moved to a few different locations whenever the company felt she was needed more elsewhere. She always dressed professionally and was very stylish for the time. She wore pantsuits, slacks with blouses or sweaters, or she had a dress on with matching shoes and handbag. Think back to the *Mary Tyler Moore Show*: that was my mother working in an office, supervising other women.

Why was it important for her to be dressed up for a job that was about bill dispatching and trucks? My mother had respect for herself and her company, took her job seriously, and was passionate about it. She felt that if you look great, you feel great. Even on weekends my mother and father dressed nicely. When my parents attended special functions, my mom would wear these long, beautiful gowns with elbow-length gloves and, of course, a matching handbag. Her influence to dress like a lady and just enjoy life was wonderful to watch and easy to absorb. She may not have purchased top-of-the-line items, but she was always well put together and looked like a million dollars.

With me tagging along, I remember my father driving my mother to someone's home where there was a full line of clothing for my mom to try on. She could choose what she liked, and she always looked beautiful. Essentially, my mom was working personally with a sales person (who today would be called a personal shopper or stylist), who either custom-ordered my mom's clothes or from whom my mom could purchase on the spot. Mom was a true shopper. She liked items unique to her so that no one else at the trucking company office or at special functions would wear the same item. I always enjoyed shopping with her because it was fun to look around. She would show me what was new and exciting, and what colors made her feel good. And I loved to go with her because, just maybe, my mom would buy something new for me.

As I grew into those awkward teenage years, playing sports was important, and I felt I knew everything there was to know about anything. I was a teenager, and teenagers know everything there is to know, right? Well, I decided to enhance my personal style while playing sports by wearing a ribbon in my hair that had to match my uniform, and my hair had to be in a perfect ponytail, and I had to have my makeup on, too. I probably looked like a . . . well, who knows what I probably looked like, but it was just my style. You can make your own conclusion—while I'm laughing about the conclusion I've come up with in my own mind. As I matured, fashion became my passion. I was still an athlete, but I decided to take some modeling classes, learn some etiquette, and became very interested in the fashion world.

My goal? Play sports, be a model, go to college, get a degree in fashion merchandising, go to work for a major retail chain, and become a buyer so that I could travel to the heart of the fashion district. During college, I worked in a small retail store to get experience and make some extra money while studying fashion merchandising. In the summertime when I'd go home, I worked two jobs to earn money for school. One job was with another retail chain, which was great experience. It was fun to help customers with their personal style by enhancing their current wardrobes.

My other job was not so glamorous. I worked in a potato chip factory! Yes, I, the fashion guru who studied fashion merchandising and who thought she had it all going on, worked in a potato chip factory. For two complete summers I worked there. Oh, how I hated it! I had a title, too: Picker, Packer, Spotter. I wanted to be in the fashion world, not the chip world. I could not help those chips.

To be honest, they were not helping my hips fit into my fashionable jeans, either. I thought, "How would Jackie Kennedy and Doris Day handle this?" As I laughed to myself, my conclusion was that Jackie Kennedy and Doris Day would not be working in a potato chip factory. Doris Day did, however, make a movie about working in a factory called *The Pajama Game*. It's a classic and, being a Doris Day fan, of course I loved it, but still I wanted to put my factory days behind me.

Every day I would show up to the factory trying to look as fashionable as I possibly could. But every day I thought to myself, "Really? It's 90 degrees outside so that means it's going to be 110 degrees inside, and there's no air conditioning. How can I look fashionable in a white smock and matching hairnet that smashes my hair down flat while I'm sweating? Where has my personal style gone?" No one cared, of course, but me. No one was allowed to wear any jewelry on their smocks to express any personality. Jewelry could fall off and then onto the conveyer belt—that would not be good.

No matter where you work or what your career, make the best of your personal style and enjoy your fashion sense whenever you can. At the potato chip factory, I made sure my shoes were appropriate and looked nice with the blue jeans I had to wear. My top was always covered by my not-so-unique nor one-of-a-kind white smock, so that didn't help much. I just kept telling myself, "I only work an eight-hour shift, and then my fashion sense will be free."

During college my mom would come to visit me for something called "Mom's Weekend." We would eat, shop, play, and shop some more. My mother spoiled me, and I was in heaven. When we weren't shopping or involved with an activity, we attended a mother's weekend luncheon and fashion show. "Oh, what fun," I thought. "This is just up my alley—fashion, fun, and food!" Every year my mom and I would go. To this day, I enjoy going to luncheons and fashion shows with her.

I have expanded this tradition of attending luncheons and fashion shows with my sister-in-law, Leslie. We seldom miss a particularly wonderful event that benefits women helping others in their community.. Some years Leslie's mother-in-law, my mom, my sister, and our aunt join us, along with many incredible women who we get to meet and become friends with. I will always treasure these afternoons as beautiful memories of sharing fashion and food.

During my junior year of college, I was elected to model in the mother's weekend show along with several other students. My practice runs and fittings for the show were truly fun, and I loved it! I was in my element and felt so passionate about who I was and what I wanted to become in my career. When I became a senior, I decided to coordinate the luncheon and fashion show with the help of other students instead of modeling.

Our show was a great success. The experience I gained to coordinate a live show was thrilling, but also nerve-racking. Right before the music began and the curtains opened, I was scared to death. Oh, what a rush! My heart was beating so fast that I was hyperventilating, and I was frantically praying that no one would fall onstage and that the music wouldn't suddenly stop. It was a successful show, and the feeling of "we did it, I did it" was incredibly awesome.

It wasn't the Super Bowl, but in my little world, it was just as big. I had wonderful choreographers, student models, and an art student so gifted and creative with backdrops and props that our show was highlighted to perfection. What an honor it was to be the general coordinator of this annual production—a lifetime memory that I will always cherish.

As my senior year was winding down, I was recruited out of college by a large retail chain for their executive training program. That company was the Bon Marché (now Macy's), and I worked for them for twelve years, in three different states and four different stores. The influence this had on me and the knowledge I gained from working at "The Bon" were priceless. At that time, we unpacked our own merchandise right there on the floor and would merchandise it for the customer. I was moving from store to store learning all about women's fashion styles and how trends would arrive in different cities at different times.

While managing different departments, I began to develop customers who would request my styling services. I kept a book on what styles certain clients liked so that I could call them to fill them in about "their" new arrivals. Having customers come in and ask for me personally and for my style guidance was thrilling, as was helping them understand the reasons why one brand worked for their body type over another or how certain colors brought out their natural glow.

While working at the Bon Marché I learned that anyone can sell just about anything as long as they can scan a barcode or punch in a UPC number into the register. But to take an item and go into different departments to pull a whole outfit together and accessorize it is the service that my clients loved and appreciated about me.

The true value that I offered my personal clients was always about them. I made sure then, and still do today, that my customers feel good about themselves and my service. I let them know that I am not judgmental, but objective. I am here to help and get to know who they are so that we as a team can find their very best looks.

A STYLISH LIFE

During my continuing life journey, I wanted to enhance my own personal style. What I found, though, is that my true passion is in helping other women discover their inner beauty so that they feel and look fabulous by projecting an image unique to their own personal style.

I found in my research that the DRES System has the best philosophy today to help my clients achieve their own beauty, balance, and confidence, inside and out. My clients need to get to know who they are first and, as confidence builds, their personal style will speak clearly about who they are before saying a single word.

When a woman lacks personal style, she also lacks confidence in who she is. Uncertainty in what to purchase can make shopping an unpleasant chore. When she lacks confidence, a woman is unbalanced and her inner beauty doesn't have a chance to shine through for others to see. She often ends up having too many items in her wardrobe that don't work well with other pieces, and then they end up sitting in the closet, sometimes with tags still attached.

MIND, BODY, AND SOUL

When you're unsure of your own personal style, you can waste hundreds, even thousands of dollars on unwise purchases. The DRES System not only helps in defining your beautiful body shape, but can also help define the fashion style you want to show off that will fit into your lifestyle.

Here are the three considerations to decide on in defining your own personal style:

Mind: What is the image I want to portray when I walk into a room? Is my beauty glowing from the inside out? Feeling beautiful on the inside shows the world that you're confident and a natural leader. The clothes you wear, your hairstyle, and how many accessories you wear all speak for you before your voice does. These things "speak" more than half of a first impression without ever saying a word. Have you heard of the expression "actions speak louder than words"? This is what a first impression is all about.

Body: "I'm worried I don't look good in the same kind of jeans my friends are wearing. Why don't these jeans look good on me? They looked so cute on my friends. I want to wear what everyone else is wearing, but I can't afford it." You might not be able to afford those jeans, but do you really want to wear everything your friends wear, anyway? Your body shape will most likely be different than your friends'. Wear clothing that best represents you and not your friends, or anyone else.

Soul: "Is this really me, and do I feel confident wearing this style? Everyone is wearing this style of pants. Is it me or am I just following a trend?" Trends come and go quickly, so you probably won't get your money's worth in a trendy item's cost per wear. No matter your body shape, you can find the best-fitting clothes when you understand your beautiful assets via the DRES System and work with them—not against them. This is a good time to ask yourself, "Is it comfortable? Do I feel confident, and is this the image I want, though I like to fit in and wear what everyone else is wearing?"

WHAT IS A PERSONAL STYLE?

Your style should be authentic and based on your personality and lifestyle traits:

Interests: What do you enjoy doing? How does this fit into your lifestyle, or how can you make it fit into your lifestyle? Do your interests make you feel good about who you are? Are you having fun when you participate in these activities, or do you just do it because it's the trend of the month? Do you include others or is it best to be alone? Whatever your interests are, make sure you are enjoying the activity that you have chosen.

Desires: Have you spent quiet time consciously deciding what you want out of life? How do you express those desires for your life? Try writing them down in a journal, which often helps you to move from thought to action. Do you use positive affirmations very often? It doesn't matter if your desires are small or large as long as they're authentic to you. Desires are goals that you haven't taken action for yet. What kind of life do you envision for yourself? What steps can you take to get to where you want to be in a year, three years, or even ten years? Write them down.

Taste: Are your tastes suitable for the lifestyle you want to live? Dress to make an impact and dress for where you want to go in your business life. Do you like to wear blinged-out jeans or classic, well-cut slacks? What are your values? These are so often reflected in a woman's style. Do your values include dressing modestly? If so, would it be appropriate to show off what you have just a little more? Make sure your style is consistent with how you want to be perceived.

Goals: Have you made a list of your goals? How often do you check them? Are your goals attainable so that you don't get too frustrated? Often breaking them down into steps, from simple to difficult, makes any goal seem more attainable. Try a realistic goal and move up to a more complicated one so that you feel the satisfaction of achievement. Goals must be believable, positive, and challenging enough to inspire you. Setting goals too high or too low could make you feel stuck and prevent your accomplishing that goal at all.

Make a checklist of your personality and lifestyle traits. Look in your closet to see if you are being authentic to yourself. Does the clothing in your closet match with your interests? If yes, then great! If not, ask yourself how you can start making a few, subtle changes. You will soon learn to love the clothing in your closet and, no matter what you choose to wear, you'll feel and look great because you understand your body shape, personal style, and your values. You will be in harmony.

A STYLE SHOULD BE APPROPRIATE

Your style should also be appropriate for the activity you're involved in. If you're going to exercise, wear clothes that fit well and are comfortable for your type of workout. Invest in good supportive shoes, too.

I teach etiquette classes, and I discuss with my students what is appropriate or inappropriate attire if they're invited to a party or another special event. I share with them the notion that style implies a degree of moral responsibility about who they are. I ask my clients about what type of party they're attending, and then they need to confirm how formal or informal the event might be. To decide on what to wear, they need to ask themselves:

- What is the weather like? Will the event be inside or outside?
- Daytime or evening?
- Does the invitation have special instructions on it?
- Who is invited? Just me or the whole family? (Always remember to RSVP within a few days.)

Here's what I ask my students, and they all cringe when I say it. Then I chuckle at the look on their faces. "Class, what would you think if you came to my etiquette class today, prepared to learn all about proper dining skills, and I greeted every one of you wearing a swimsuit?"

They all look at me and say, "Ewww! No way, that's too much for my eyes." I laugh and tell them that I may be comfortable and confident in how I look in my swimsuit, but is it respectful to be teaching manners with not much on? If this happened to me, I would be thinking, "Is this instructor for real?! I just can't take this teacher seriously because of what they are wearing—or not wearing."

The same goes for business attire. Make sure you are appropriate and dressed for success with a touch of your own personality added. Accessories are a perfect way to show your personal style through your handbag, shoes, jewelry, and eyewear. Keep your accessories simple, clean, and classic. If you like to wear a piece of trendy jewelry with a splash of color, this is a great way to express yourself. Watch out for accessories that make noise, though. You don't want to be heard five cubicles away.

As another example, when attending a funeral, you might ask yourself what to wear. Most people choose a dark color for mourning, but the only little black dress you have in your closet is a cocktail dress. You know it fits and looks great on you, but is the style what you want to portray at this event? Your little black dress is a sleeveless shift cut short above the knees, with a low neckline and a slit up the side that shows quite a bit of leg. Okay, okay, yes, you look hot. This little black dress is perfect for a red carpet runway event, but not so much for a funeral.

For a serious occasion like this, think about the style required for the event you are attending. Your style is about who you are, but you still need to dress for the occasion and be appropriate. Yes, it's important to dress in your fashion style so that you can connect with the image you want to convey. But remember, remember, remember! Dress appropriately for the occasion so you're showing respect for yourself and others.

THE IMPORTANCE OF YOUR PERSONAL STYLE

Why is it important to develop your own personal fashion style? Simply stated, it makes you look and feel brilliant. Your inner beauty comes out and shines brightly when you feel and look great. It may take some time to develop your personal style, but you will get there. Buy the best quality you can afford; it's important to look your best. Also ask yourself, "Would I wear this because my friends are wearing it or because it's truly me?" A style is about expressing your individuality through your clothes. Style defines you.

You may love to wear dark colors, but maybe you're also drawn to the color orange. I say, mix and match them. Try on three or four fun bracelets in different shades of orange. The goal is to make sure your accessories align with your style. If your style for the office is a classic corporate look, make sure your accessories match that style. For example, an ethnic, bohemian-style bracelet will most likely clash if your style is a classic corporate look. Try to remember that each element should be consistent with your style; otherwise, they may look wrong when matched together.

As we age, our personal style may slightly change, too. If you strive for a timeless beauty, that is a great look! Make sure it's not an era-specific (and thus dated) style that you get stuck in. Think about how funny someone would look dressed now in a 1980s' Boy George look! Take a look at old magazines to see what was in style then, and then look in magazines of today. The designs of timeless pieces may have changed slightly, but the lines are still the same style. Being timeless is very fashionable.

For me it was all about ribbons in my hair and then barrettes, as I entered my teens. As an adult, I still wear barrettes or claw clips (so can you). I make sure they're age-appropriate and consistent with the look and style I want to achieve. I enjoy having my hair curled for a soft look, which is much more age-appropriate for me and my style than matching colored ribbons.

If you dress sloppily in the professional world, you're perceived as being a generally sloppy person. What do your office and your desk look like? You may lose credibility with coworkers or clients if your desk is a mess. When reaching into your handbag and pulling out an item, is it crazy with a cascade of items falling out everywhere? What does your car look like when you're driving a client to lunch? These are all nonverbal ways of communication. Make sure you are communicating the right message.

YOUR PERSONAL STYLE GOAL: THE UNIQUE EXPRESSION OF YOU!

How do you want to be perceived? What desire or image do you want to project? Developing your personal fashion style is a lifelong journey and not necessarily a destination. Figure out who and what you are all about—take notes! Cut out pictures from magazines and ask yourself:

- What are your fashion likes and dislikes?
- What looks and feels great on your body shape?
- What colors make you feel good when you wear them?
- What do you struggle with? Accessorizing, selecting colors, or outfit styling? Have your stylist help with your struggles.

Fashion requires money, just as your own signature style requires self-awareness, confidence, personality, and creativeness. Style equals your individuality, and a signature style is that unique touch you're known for. Your signature style is also your overall look on how you put it all together, e.g., a flower on your lapel, a bright handbag you carry, or a certain way you tie your scarf.

Questions from My Clients

Q: I really love this skirt, but does it really look good on me?

A: First, I ask my client to try on the skirt. If it's a good fit, then I'll check the length. I'll adjust it to show the difference a skirt's length makes, either shorter or longer. Sometimes, that's all that is needed. I recommend everyone have a good tailor who really understands garment fitting.

Q: I don't have anything to go with these pants, but I can't seem to part with them.
A: As a stylist, I would look into their accessories. If they have scarves, I pick one that goes with the pants. Then I'd choose a basic, solid-color blouse or sweater in a harmonizing style and color; then they have a whole new look! My clients and I address the questions together and decide what best fits the client's personal style and lifestyle.

Q: I have so many separates because I usually buy clothing at sales. But then nothing goes together!
A: I have helped clients put outfits together that they never would have even thought of putting together. I've shown them how to add a scarf to a dress that might not be the best color for them, but the dress fits well. By putting the scarf up closer to the face, the dress's color is no longer a concern, and they look amazing! My goal for my clients is to always enhance their beauty and their assets.

MISTAKES WE ALL MAKE

These are some of the typical things that happen to women if they have never used or been helped by a stylist:

- *Have you ever bought something and never worn it?* Why is that? Is it the wrong color? Remember, color is very important to enhance your natural glow. If you wear the correct color, you will feel vibrant and look healthy. If the wrong color is next to your skin, you may look dull, tired, and shadows will appear.
- *"Why is it that the item I just purchased looked good on the mannequin in the store but not on me at home?"* Most mannequins are made to resemble a fit model. Having a tailor is very important.

No one has the perfect fit model shape. Having a tailor can help save those items in your closet with a little alteration.

- *Have you ever looked in your closet and said, "I have nothing to wear"?* I would ask if your clothing no longer fits or if it's time to edit your personal style and closet. The average woman wastes over half of every dollar on unwise or impulse purchases. Whatever has frustrated you in the past, I believe that once you learn how to shop for your body shape and you know what to look for, shopping will become enjoyable, quickly—and your dollars will be wisely spent.
- *"I can never find anything when I need it."* Make sure you are looking for your item during the right season. If you like to shop at off-season sales or outlet stores, keep and bring with you an ongoing list of needed items. Also make sure you are shopping in the proper stores for your personal style and lifestyle.
- *"I'm not sure if I'm getting an honest opinion on how an item really looks on me before I buy it."* It's always helpful to have your DRES System Stylist along to guide you in your purchases. Once you have gained confidence, making decisions will be easier, and you will naturally select items that will best suit your body shape.
- *"It takes too long."* With understanding of your personal style and proper fit, shopping will become quick and enjoyable.
- *"I can't find my size, so I compromise when it comes to fashion."* If your size is not on the floor, be sure to ask the sales person. Sometimes stores don't display every item in every size and might be able to obtain it elsewhere. Remember: if you don't love it, don't buy it.
- *"All I can find right now is this fashion trend and it doesn't look good on me."* Make sure that the stores where you're shopping carry fashion styles you want or need, and that the store fits your lifestyle, too.
- *"I'm unhappy with my weight and body shape, so I dread shopping."* No matter your shape, size, or age, love who you are and enhance your best assets so that you always look and feel brilliant.

- *"There's always low lighting, a limited number of items to try on, and no sales help."* This truly can be frustrating when there is no sales help to be found. So many stores have turned to a central checkout spot, and sales help has been cut. Bringing your stylist along to help you shop can and will save you time and money.

To build a personal style, you must first identify your beautiful gem shape from the DRES System. My clients' style is all about individuality and expressing who they are. I am here to guide them with my expertise and to build their confidence within themselves. In working with the DRES System fashion styles, I help my clients relate these to their own personal styles. The work we do together ultimately should reflect the image that they would like to project and that they feel most comfortable with for their lifestyle.

YOUR VERY OWN SIGNATURE STYLE: WHAT IS IT?

A signature style is an outfit you wear and is unique to you, like the ribbons in my hair that had to perfectly match my uniform for my sporting events when I was younger. Christina Aguilera's platinum-blond hair and bright red lips would be her signature style. Lady Gaga wears costumes onstage unique to her. A few other signature styles are Sarah Palin's stylish eyewear and updo. Michelle Obama's signature style is a belted waist to show off her figure, and she tends to wear long, open jackets. Barbara Bush: Do you remember her signature style? Yes, it would be her beautiful pearls that she always wears.

Why is a signature style important? These styles identify each individual in her own way—it is who they are. Their signature style fits with their lifestyle and portrays what they want to project. It showcases their inner beauty to the outside for all to see.

Why does anyone have a signature style? To show a piece of who that person is and let their personality shine. A signature style makes my clients feel confident in themselves and shows what they're made of. My mother likes butterflies. When I see a scarf or piece of jewelry that has a butterfly on it, I think of her.

Do you wear a big, bold ring on your index finger, a beautiful vintage piece that was passed down from your grandmother? Or is it something simple like wearing your hair in a ponytail? Whatever your signature style may be, just make sure it is authentic to you and your life.

YOUR IMAGE SPEAKS FOR YOU

How important is your personal image? First impressions are very important, so make sure your personal style is speaking correctly.

When I met my late husband, Matt, in college, he was so cute and shy, and a muscular athlete. He majored in exercise and physiology. I was a student in the College of Home Economics, with an emphasis in fashion merchandising. I looked at this great hunk and said to myself, "His eyes are beautiful, his smile contagious, but oh, my gosh! What is he wearing?!"

Now don't call me a snob, but how could I date someone who had no fashion sense? He was a U.S. Marine who was always wearing camouflage pants with a sweatshirt (and not his uniform), or he was wearing shorts, which, back in the day, were short-shorts, with a sweatshirt and white, mid-calf socks. Was he crazy? He thought he looked very stylish and felt very confident in his own personal style. I had to smile because I, on the other hand, was in my beautiful angora sweater with matching cords and boots. No ribbon in my hair—I had moved up to barrettes. Matt still won my heart. It must have been his smile, his eyes, and his charm—because I know it wasn't his fashion sense. As we kept dating each other through college, I took Matt on as my personal project.

I showed him how to enjoy his wardrobe but be more fashionable, with his own sense of personal style so that he could still feel confident yet comfortable. After college we married and, every so often, we would look through our college photos and chuckle because of our fashion styles: Matt in his shorts and sweatshirts, and me, all put together in my fashionable outfits. I loved him for who he was, and Matt caught on when it was appropriate to wear his shorts with mid-calf socks versus when he needed to wear a more fashionable outfit. Once he graduated from college and started his career, and had to wear a suit every day, he looked sharp and felt confident because he had found an image and style that enhanced his personality. His mind, body, and soul were in sync.

TWO TYPES OF COMMUNICATION: VERBAL AND NONVERBAL

Verbal: what you say. And nonverbal: what you do and wear. Your visual presence speaks much louder than what you say. One study at UCLA indicated that up to 93 percent of communication effectiveness is determined by nonverbal cues. Even though your words make a smaller impression, make sure the volume, tone, and pitch of your voice are professional. If you are wearing a high-end business suit and look very powerful, but when speaking your voice is squeaky and high-pitched, your credibility is lost. It is important to know which clothes enhance your assets; the image you want to project is a whole package, voice and all.

As verbal communication is not a high percentage of your first impression, posture plays a large part in your nonverbal image: 38 percent. So by standing tall, you look confident and you will also look as though you are ten pounds lighter. Good posture can also alleviate back pain, headaches, and even leg pain. Posture is very important to everyone's well being and, by practicing great posture habits, your clothes will fit and look so good on you that you'll feel better, too.

Undergarments are also very important to style and image. To look your best, purchase supportive and well-made undergarments. They help clothes fit better and help prevent unintentionally showing too much cleavage or visible panty lines, for instance.

Again, the way you look reflects on the way you feel, act, and conduct yourself. And that can change the way others respond and react toward you.

IMAGE: APPROACHABLE AND PROFESSIONAL

How can you take someone seriously if they don't act professionally? This really goes back to first impressions and how one is perceived. As someone who has studied etiquette and is a certified etiquette instructor, I express the importance of business etiquette to my clients and guide them on how kindness and self-respect as well as respect for others and their property are the true foundations of manners. If my clients do not understand the importance of manners and they are in the professional world, this could make or break a deal at a lunch meeting. A meal is about conversation and relationships, not just shoveling in food. Your image is important as a whole package. It's not just about what you're wearing.

If you talk with a mouthful of food, others may not want to eat with you or they may feel you aren't the best candidate to professionally represent them, for example. Below are some suggested tips about good business manners:

- When meeting someone for the first time, stand up tall, use good eye contact, and repeat the person's name to make them feel good and help you to remember it. Extend your hand and offer a firm handshake to that person. The best tip? Be a good listener—show interest in the person you have just met.
- Learn basic dining table etiquette, like water and wine glass placement, which fork is used first, and what to do (or not do)

with your napkin. Know who is paying the bill before the meal begins, and if there are any special dietary needs.

- Should you floss your teeth at the table because you have food stuck in between your teeth? No. How about ordering a dessert to go when you aren't paying the bill? No. Buffet lines: Should you show up starving and go through the line five times? No. These probably seem like no-brainers, but some adults just don't know how to handle a business lunch or dinner. And keep the conversation to business rather than your personal life, unless you're invited to share something—and keep it appropriate to the occasion.

Remember: It's the whole package of what you are wearing, what your posture says, what and how you relate to others, and the tone of your voice that makes you approachable yet professional.

When wearing an item that harmonizes with your DRES Profile and your DRES System forty-two Ultimate Colors Palette, and you are showing your best assets, you will look and feel confident, you will stand and walk taller, and you will be perceived as a leader. If you want to be a leader and move up in your company, spend what time you can with people who are in those higher-up positions. Your impressions count verbally and nonverbally.

For instance, when you walk into a room looking sharp, polished, and ready to engage with others, they will respond to you positively. They'll want to get to know you, and you will be making it clear that you want to know more about them. Your clothing, style, and genuine interest in other people allow them to perceive you as approachable, confident, trustworthy, and even powerful. Pulling your style and image together will give you more career opportunities because you come across as being passionate in your line of work, and in life.

If your image is confident, polite, and approachable, I can almost guarantee that you will be successful because people will respond to you in kind and will want to learn from you. Civility is always a great trait and makes your personal image shine.

NOT WORKING IN AN OFFICE?

Say you are not a professional working in an office, but someone who works from home or you are a stay-at-home mom. You might think, "I don't go anywhere, so why dress nicely? And why would I want to dress up for the kids or while I make telephone calls from my kitchen table?"

First, always dress up for yourself—you're worth it! Those working from home show great self-discipline, and stay-at-home moms have one of the most important and most difficult jobs around. Dressing appropriately for your day shows your self-respect, and teaches children the importance of that self-respect in many ways. One day you may want to return to working outside the home or transition back to working in an office instead of at home. It will be an easier transition if you stay in touch with your personal style and have the appropriate wardrobe already available.

MAKE THE MOST OF YOUR STYLE

There are components that will help you enhance and maximize your personal style. Buy a few fashion-related and women's magazines. Look at all the outfits on the models to see what appeals to you.

"Fashion is what you wear; style is how you wear it."
—Author unknown

True Color: Your DRES Stylist can help create your forty-two Ultimate Colors Palette, unique to you. Do you have a warm or cool undertone? This is important so that the colors you wear enhance your natural glow. There is a color that looks good on most women, no matter their undertone. That color is turquoise. However, the colors black and white tend to only look good on less than 5 percent of women.

Black absorbs light while white reflects it. Black can look very slimming and elegant, but it's unflattering worn next to most complexions. Black can be aging as it spotlights fatigue, wrinkles, and shadows. Wearing a scarf or bright jewelry around your face is a great way to enjoy wearing black. Since white reflects light, this color can make everything appear larger. Break up whites by adding a touch of color with a scarf around your waist as a belt and neutral, open-toed shoes. This will give you a fresh, light, and fun look.

CHOOSE A FASHION STYLE

Developing your fashion style takes time. It's a journey that everyone can enjoy. Choosing a fashion style is all about who and what you are and what your life is all about. You wear an item because it feels right and lets your inner beauty shine.

Sometimes a signature style finds you in an item or color that you don't even think about. You just love it, wear it often, and it becomes a natural part of you and your style. A great example would be when a friend calls on the phone and says, "I thought of you today. I saw this hot-pink Kate Spade handbag in a boutique, and it made me want to call you."

So a signature style may be as simple as a particular color or handbag style or a fragrance. Whatever it may be, it's your signature, and it makes people think of you. Learn to love your DRES Body Shape. No matter if you're a Diamond, Ruby, Emerald, or Sapphire, embracing your best assets can save you time and money. Embracing your shape will cause your confidence to grow and help make you feel and look beautiful.

Your DRES Stylist can help you find your best style, create a DRES System StyleLog or an online DRESbook. A DRES StyleLog is a photo catalog of all your own best outfits, complete with accessories. This offers such an easy way to keep track of your personal style. Plus, you can clip or snap pictures from your favorite fashion magazines and use them for future shopping dates with your DRES System Personal Stylist. A DRES StyleLog is a wonderful way to itemize and categorize your outfits for work, formal occasions, and every day in between.

YOUR PERSONAL STYLE BOOK

The online DRES Club Profile is another wonderful tool to use. You can shop online with your DRES Stylist and figure out what items will be best for you. This is a tool to guide you where to shop for your DRES Gem Body Shape, plus you can talk with your stylist online for help. Once again, clip photos from magazines. Don't overthink it; just cut and set aside to share with your personal stylist later.

QUALITY OR QUANTITY

As I was growing up, quantity seemed to be more important than quality. As a young adult, I had five pink blouses. I liked all of them, but I was only wearing two of them. I wore these two over and over because they felt good, their shades of pink were just right, and their fit was perfect. Those other blouses stayed in the closet and were never worn. Add up their cost and that is a lot of wasted money.

In helping women edit their closets, a DRES System Stylist is objective in looking over each wardrobe. We tend to be emotionally attached to our clothing, so as a DRES System client, you have total control of keeping or parting with items in your closet.

As a DRES Stylist, I can be as gentle or as direct as you want me to be when it comes to edits. Clothing items often have a story behind them, such as a memory about when it was worn (think senior prom dress) or that it is a sentimental piece passed down from a relative. The psychology of attachment could be a whole different chapter.

That's where I can be objective, not judgmental, and help guide you in your decision of what to do with an item. What I've learned over the years and I now teach my client is to purchase quality. It is much better than quantity. My goal as my client is for you to love every piece in your closet; you will want to wear anything you choose from your closet over and over again. When you find good quality on sale, that's a bonus; every woman loves a good deal. Looking for a deal is fun and definitely beneficial, but don't buy it just because it was on sale.

COST PER WEAR: DIAMONDS VS. A TRENDY JACKET

Which one would you invest in? I would like both, please! There are questions my clients need to ask themselves, and they need to be aware of price. To calculate out what the cost per wear is going to be on an item is important and worth the knowledge.

Cost per wear = cost of garment ÷ the number of times you'll wear it

Take the diamond earrings (please!). The range of the cost varies greatly depending on cut, color, clarity, and carat. Let's just say for easy math that the earrings cost $1,000. Your trendy jacket costs $400.

Cost per wear for earrings: $1,000.00 ÷ 100 = $10.00
Cost per wear for jacket: $400.00 ÷ 3 = $133.00

So you can see that this is a simple formula. The idea is to show the cost per wear over a period of time and how quality can be cost-efficient compared to something trendy. Budget is also a huge factor in my client's wardrobe. You need to consider your budget before making any purchases. High cost-per-wear items include a wedding dress, trendy items, and a bridesmaid dress. Low cost-per-wear items include jeans, diamond earrings, and mid-heel pumps for work. Try out new things, certainly, but make sure the item you purchase fits your lifestyle, too. Otherwise, you won't feel comfortable in it, and it will sit in your closet as an unwise purchase.

FIT AND COLOR

When I started modeling years ago, I did both still photography and runway work. I later tried video, which was different due to camera angles, microphones, and lighting. When you model for a camera versus an audience, the camera's eye is different than the human eye. As a model, you need to make sure that the fit of clothes is perfect for the body shape, the lights, and the angles.

While modeling, I need to make sure that my clothes and the color I am wearing are correct for a healthy glow, especially in commercials. Light reflects differently with different colors, patterns, and angles. I need to make sure the creases of a garment do not shadow in the camera. I make sure my pose is at a stance that is the most flattering view for my shape, and I make sure the sound of my voice is appropriate. Today, it is much easier for film and camera to be manipulated with color, lighting, and Photoshop. But I still need to be at my best in what I am wearing and how the garment fits, along with how I am posed.

As for runway modeling, the garment I'm modeling needs to fit my body shape to enhance my assets to their fullest. When I'm wearing the right color and style, my look harmonizes and I feel like a million bucks. I also enjoy and feel the excitement of the audience enjoying the outfits that I am modeling. You might be thinking to yourself, "You are a model; you can wear anything."

Everyone, including models, feels they have flaws and areas of their bodies that they would like to conceal. With the help of your DRES System Personal Stylist, you can learn the difference between how a garment fits your body shape and how certain lines give the illusion of a fabulous figure. When you are wearing the correct color, fit, and style, your best assets are being highlighted, and you too will be in harmony and feel like a million bucks!

Why hire a DRES Stylist to help guide you to make efficient and wise purchases for your personal style? There are a variety of reasons women request my services as a DRES System Personal Stylist. Some women feel stuck in their fashion style, while some would like to refine their image due to a promotion. Others just want help with closet editing because their careers are changing, or they are retiring, or returning to the workforce.

Having a personal stylist can direct you to the correct path for success. Your stylist can save you time and guide you where to shop, so shopping becomes enjoyable and quick. As a stylist, I can also help educate you to shop wisely and, when you understand your personal fashion style, your shopping will harmonize with your lifestyle. I am here to help, not judge—and you will learn to do more with less. I can guide you in what to wear and when to wear it so that you will look and feel confident and project a brilliant image. I will also help you to understand what colors look best on you and what style is the best fit for your body shape.

Remember, ladies: the most important thing about your new look is to be true to yourself. At the same time, a new personal style can make you look and feel brilliant from the inside out. If you feel good, you will shine, and people around you will notice and compliment you on how great you look in that particular color or style of jacket. You will be perceived as confident, and others will want to get to know who you are. People will want to be around you because whatever you're doing is working, so your brilliance is positive and contagious.

One of my goals for you as my client would be that you love every item you have in your wardrobe. You will want to wear every item over and over again because it will represent your personal style, be authentic to you, and fit perfectly with your lifestyle.

I hope that my passions for fashion and image combine to help all of my clients feel comfortable, because you inspire me. When my clients better understand how they would like to portray themselves through their image and lifestyle choices, they succeed at being approachable, professional, and successful individuals. And I know that, in helping my clients discover their personal style, they also find their inner confidence.

Your image is part of your personal style—make a great first impression. Enjoy your personal style! It is who you are and is meant to help you live life to its fullest.

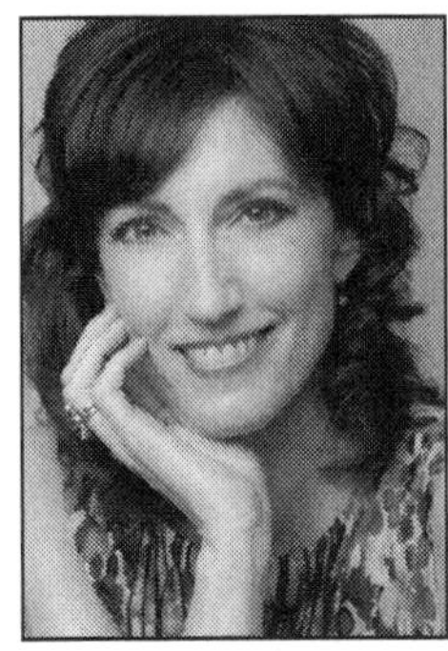

Lori Goddard-Weed

DRES System–Certified Personal Stylist

Image Is It
www.holobi.com/lorg
Imageisit@gmail.com
Everett, Washington

Lori earned her bachelor of science degree from Oregon State University (OSU). Her emphasis was fashion merchandising and business administration. She was active in the Greek system, and served as standards chairman for her sorority, Alpha Gamma Delta. She also represented OSU Panhellenic as a rush counselor. Lori was also honored as first runner-up in a Miss OSU Contest.

She specializes in enhancing personal style and image. She is also certified in wardrobe edits, makeup application, accessorizing, and etiquette. She started her own business, Image Is It. As a DRES System-Certified Stylist, she helps guide clients to enhance their beautiful assets so that they can shine from the inside out. Lori is also a certified etiquette instructor with Final Touch Finishing School, and teaches classes year-round for adults and children. Lori feels that personal style and image are a perfect combination for success.

Lori stays involved with fashion and image by continuing to model for print, runway, and television commercials. She has been a skin care consultant for the past sixteen years with a top cosmetics company. Lori also enjoys being involved with civic duties as a volunteer for "Queen, It's a New Day," a two-day makeover event for abused and battered women. She also works with the YMCA to help raise money to brighten the future of America's children, and volunteers in her hometown's public school system.

When not working with clients, Lori enjoys spending time with her husband and four boys. She loves to ski and garden.

CHAPTER 5

EDITING

LESS IS ENOUGH

By Colleen Bradley

What do you call it when you know and love your body exactly as it is today, wear only what you're totally comfortable in—outfits designed to accentuate your best features, and leave the house every day feeling like a million bucks? It's called *signature style*.

Would you like to be able to dress for any occasion with complete confidence? How about knowing how to dress for your specific lifestyle? The reality is that we wear 20 percent of our wardrobes 80 percent of the time, wasting hundreds of dollars on clothing that we will never wear. Does this sound familiar?

- You find yourself looking in your closet and seeing clothing with the price tags still attached, yet to be worn?
- You have multiple sizes of jeans or pants hanging in your closet, hoping to lose that infamous last five pounds?
- You find yourself with an overabundance of black and white clothing?
- You struggle with dressing age-appropriately while retaining your sense of style?
- You find yourself spending the entire day in your workout clothing because it's easier than figuring out what to wear?
- You want to incorporate trends into your wardrobe but don't know how to make them work?

Every day we get up and decide what to wear. Often this creates great stress for us rather than providing us with a creative way to express ourselves. When you feel great and look your best, it influences your mindset for the day, giving you that extra spring in your step and boost in your confidence. I believe the best thing you can wear is confidence.

Your DRES System Personal Stylist will give you the tools and knowledge to bring out your personal brilliance so that you can improve the way you view your body image and wardrobe. We all possess a unique beauty and authentic style. It's our goal to bring out that beauty for the world to see. So let's get started.

Using a three-step wardrobe editing process, you will wake up to a closet full of clothes that you love to wear, make better decisions when shopping and, best of all, stay true to yourself with a renewed sense of confidence. After this process, what you reach for in your closet will be flattering, stylish, and a reflection of your personality. Getting ready for any occasion will be a fun, stress-free experience. The DRES System will provide you with the organizational tips and tricks to optimize your closet space. It begins with the right tools and supplies.

ORGANIZING CHECKLIST

Choosing the Right Hanger

Just like your clothing, your closet needs to start off with a strong foundation. A key element for that foundation is your hangers. I know you might be hesitant to purchase hangers versus keeping your existing hangers but, I assure you, you will thank me for this recommendation. I have never yet had a client who hasn't been amazed by the impact this simple change makes in their closet. Not only do the right hangers save space and prevent clothing items from slipping off and getting lost in the bottom of your closet, but they instantly provide a clearer picture of your wardrobe: your eyes see the clothes and not the chaos of a mismatched collection of wire and plastic hangers. My favorites are called Huggable Hangers®. They are a skinny, nonslip, velvet-covered hanger. You can find a less expensive version of this type of hanger at Costco. Your goal: to have as much of your wardrobe hanging as is possible, except for pieces that could become stretched out or misshapen.

The Beauty of the Digital Camera

When it comes to creating your ultimate wardrobe, a picture is worth a thousand words. For example, have you ever looked back at old photos and thought, "What was I thinking? That looks terrible!" Working with your DRES System Personal Stylist can prevent this from ever happening again.

With today's wonderful digital cameras, it's easier than ever for your personal stylist to take pictures of you in your outfits and then evaluate them on a computer screen. This will allow you and your personal stylist to honestly critique the coordinated look. The camera does not lie. It is important to be wearing the complete outfit when photographed versus just displaying the outfit on flat surface, so you can see the true three-dimensional result. You can visually determine if the fit, proportion, color, and accessories are in harmony with your body type and with each other.

You and your personal stylist will consider these factors when looking at your photos:

- **Fit:** Is your clothing lying properly against your body or is something too snug, too loose, too short, or too long?
- **Proportion:** Does the combination of what you have on create balance for your body type? Does it make you look taller or shorter, heavier or thinner? Is it cutting your body in half or drawing your eye down, rather than toward your face?
- **Color:** Does the color make your skin and eyes look bright or dull? Does it overpower or complement you?
- **Accessories:** Are they in scale with your size so they complete your look? Or do they overwhelm you, creating visual overload?

Getting the Total Look with a Full-Length Mirror

For the times when you don't have your personal stylist helping you, a full-length mirror is the next best thing. A basic full-length mirror should be at least forty-eight inches tall. This length will enable you to view yourself in full height by standing a few feet from the mirror.

Beware: not all mirrors are created equal. A less-expensive mirror could more likely negatively distort your true reflection. It's worth spending a few extra dollars for a higher-quality mirror. When putting together your best looks, it's important to see your full body (including footwear) to make sure that you've gotten the proportions correct for your figure. The only way to do this is to put on the entire outfit head to toe, including accessories. Over time and after working with your personal stylist, you'll feel more confident and comfortable putting together outfits that complement you. What stands between you and looking fabulous are some tough decisions. The results are worth it. Great wardrobes don't just happen. They take time and planning.

Although cleaning out your closet can be an overwhelming task, there are plenty of benefits. This process will help you get organized and reacquaint you with everything in your wardrobe.

Donation or Sorting Bags

For your wardrobe edit, you will need to designate sorting piles. This can be done simply by using the space on your bed or floor. When it's determined that an item is not staying in your closet, we will move it to one of the following piles:

- Donations
- Dry cleaning
- Consignment
- Alterations
- Off-season
- Sentimental
- Too small
- Too large

CLARITY IN YOUR CLOSET

Do you know what's in your closet? Do you feel stuck in a style rut by wearing the same outfits because it's easier and more comfortable than having to navigate your closet and create a new look? Let's break out of that rut and create clarity in your closet! A wardrobe and closet edit can help you rediscover your clothing options and put together a strategic plan to fill the voids. The final result is a focused, organized, and an "easy-to-shop" collection in your closet. After this process, you will see great and unexpected ways to maximize what you already have in your wardrobe. It's time to stop procrastinating, get reacquainted with your clothing, and get editing. You'll feel great when it's done!

Clothing Edit by Season

My family and I have lived in Austin, Texas, for the past seven years. Unlike where I grew up in Ohio, I have found that Texas really has only two seasons in relation to clothing options for the majority of the year, whereas in Ohio, we enjoyed a true spring, summer, fall, and winter. Where you live will help you determine how to sort your clothing and footwear by season. The other critical factor is storage space. If you have the ability to separate and store your off-season clothing elsewhere, that is ideal. If space is limited, just group together the off-season items and put them toward the back of your closet.

Off-Season Clothing Care

In creating a less stressful experience for you while getting ready in the morning, it's important to have easy access to items that you can wear for the current season and not have your closet filled with things that are out of season. By having only the current season choices at your fingertips, you will save time and frustration while getting dressed every day.

We all invest significantly in our wardrobes, so it's important to properly care and store your clothing to protect your investment. Nothing is more heartbreaking than to discover your favorite jacket has been a gourmet lunch for moths over the winter or that a stain on your blouse is now permanent because it was stored dirty. Here are a few important tips about proper long-term care and storage for your off-season clothing:

- Never store items in dry-cleaning bags. All clothing should be removed from the clear plastic bags as soon as you get home. Plastic bags inhibit the fabric from breathing and can promote the formation of mildew and cause fume fading. Fume fading will yellow whites and discolor colored garments.
- Hang your clothes on proper hangers to help maintain their shape. Take a moment to button or zip items. The nicer they're stored on the hanger, the nicer they will look when you pull them out to wear them again.
- Get a canvas garment-storage bag. This will protect suits, dresses, and jackets from dust, while allowing fabrics to breathe. Leather is susceptible to drying and cracking if kept in plastic.
- Keep sweaters folded. Sweaters can quickly lose their shape if kept on a hanger. If you do not have space to stack them, keep them folded over a hanger.
- Use cedar hanger inserts. Cedar offers protection from moth and mildew damage.
- Never store dirty clothing. Deodorant and other stains can become permanent if stored over long periods of time.
- Store tall boots with boot shaper inserts. This will help keep the shape of your boots and keep them looking new.

YOUR IDEAL WARDROBE

Your ideal wardrobe is waiting for you. We can look at magazines or in store window displays and desire that gorgeous handbag, perfect pair of jeans, or beautiful dress, and think, "That's my dream piece!" The challenge comes when we finally have it but don't know what to wear it with, or have no event to wear it for, or it just doesn't look like we thought it would when we try it on at home. Your ideal wardrobe can be a reality when you have a closet filled with items that work for your body type, coloring, proportion, and lifestyle. The goal is to have great looks available within your closet to meet any of your activities each day.

By working with a DRES System Personal Stylist, you will learn which key silhouettes, fabrics, and colors will flatter and enhance your particular coloring and body type. Knowledge is power, and it's very beneficial when building the best selections for a basic wardrobe. It's about having the right items in your wardrobe at all times.

Although we all have specific clothing needs that vary based on lifestyle, all of us want to feel prepared when the unexpected happens. Far too often we have something come up in our lives, whether it be a sudden interview, dinner, work function or business trip, and we panic. We head to our closets and think, "What on earth am I going to wear?" Typically, the next step in our panicked state is to head to a store and make an impulsive purchase on something that's less than great. In the end, we have wasted time, money, and energy, and still didn't look or feel our best. That can change, and it all begins with the DRES Profile and wardrobe edit.

Lifestyle Needs

In the wardrobe editing process, your unique profile is created by discussing what takes place during a typical week in your life. Your personal stylist will learn about your life, including how you spend your time during the weekdays and weekends. In conjunction with that, we determine the fashion style that best fits your personality. Our goal is to define your personal style statement. This is a combination of how you would like to be perceived and the image you want to project. The amount of time spent in the following clothing categories will determine how to shape your wardrobe during the edit.

- **Formal:** Occasions and events requiring a long gown, cocktail dress, or evening wear.
- **Work:** Based on your career clothing needs, items that will be worn to work.

- **Dress-Casual:** For events like weekend office meetings, lunches with friends, date nights, or volunteer functions.
- **Casual:** Everyday dressing in a non-work environment.
- **Active:** Clothing based on your workout and fitness activities.

A review of your lifestyle needs will uncover areas that are lacking or have gaps. For example, I have a client who recently moved from California to Texas. She owns a marketing company, based in California, where she previously went into an office each day. After her relocation to Texas, she has continued to run her California office, but remotely. The change of working from an office each day in California into a home-based office in Texas created a significant shift in her lifestyle. It became obvious that she needed more focus on casual and dress-casual clothing, rather than suits and formal work clothing. She described her need to me as, "I need everyday clothes that I would feel good to be seen in." She wanted stylish looks a step above workout clothing, but nothing too fussy. While running errands or grocery shopping, if she ran into a friend, she wanted to feel good about how she looked.

USING YOUR DRES BODY SHAPE WHILE EDITING

After working with your personal stylist, and keeping the DRES Profile in mind as you go through your closet, you will have the tools and knowledge to understand why an item looks fantastic on you or is less than great. Embracing your Diamond, Ruby, Emerald or Sapphire DRES Body Shape and working with it will help tremendously.

The illustrated DRES System StyleGuide will help you find the best fit and balance for your shape. As you edit your clothing, you can focus on the silhouette and shape of the item and remove those items that don't fit your profile. The DRES StyleGuide provides you with valuable tips on every aspect of your wardrobe including necklines, skirt lengths, sleeves, and bodice length for your jackets.

For example, I have a client who would get fit-frustrated because she has wider hips and a smaller waist. Most of her pants have to be altered for them to fit properly. It doesn't matter if her weight fluctuates up or down—the width of her bone structure in her hips doesn't change. So once you learn how to dress your shape, you can use your DRES StyleGuide to provide tips on what to look for based on your individual shape.

MAKING THE CUT

Why is it that getting dressed in the morning is so often a difficult and frustrating experience? If you are like most of us, you stare at a closet full of clothing, including items you never wear: bargains you just couldn't pass up or things you hope to wear if you could only lose those last few pounds. Getting dressed has become a very negative and exasperating way to start your day. Once your wardrobe is organized and categorized, you will have a new perspective, along with a boost to your confidence, and will be very glad you did so.

After a recent wardrobe edit, my client said that she now wakes up excited about getting dressed in the mornings. She opens her closet knowing that everything fits and is flattering. Her closet is now full of possibilities instead of potential disappointment.

Together with your DRES System Personal Stylist, you can create new outfits from your existing wardrobe, plus incorporate accessories and the season's most fun trends to refresh your look.

It's A Keeper!

One of the things I love about doing wardrobe edits with my clients is discovering the unexpected. It's like a fantastic treasure hunt and a walk down memory lane combined into one adventure. It's common to feel a bit apprehensive about having someone in your closet and to worry that they will tell you to get rid of all your clothes, but I assure you, that's not the case. What's more common is the discovery of all the great pieces hidden away that you've forgotten you had, never knew what to wear with, or just needed a little updating from a fresh perspective. As we evaluate each piece, here is the checklist used to determine if "It's a Keeper." We need to be able to answer yes to all of the following questions:

- Is it a good color for your skin tone?
- Does it fit your fashion style and lifestyle needs?
- Is it right for your DRES Gem Body Shape and proportions?
- Is it the right size for you exactly as your body is today?
- Have you worn it in the last six to twelve months? If not, why?
- Is it in good condition?

Knowing that we women wear only 20 percent of our clothing 80 percent of the time, you will benefit more from having a smaller selection of fabulous choices rather than from a closetful of mediocrity. You deserve to have clothes you love to wear and make you feel good when you wear them.

What Was I Thinking?

As you continue to evaluate each item in your wardrobe, it's inevitable that you will come across those items that just make you laugh out loud. It could be something from a distant decade, or something that you just have no idea why you were inspired to spend your hard-earned dollars on and it's been hanging in your closet ever since, gathering dust. The good news is that one woman's fashion fiasco is another's dream find. There are plenty of wonderful organizations where you may donate those items and give someone else the chance to love them. I know when I left corporate America, I donated my suits to Dress for Success, and it felt great. Pick an organization that you would like to support and feel good about giving back to. I promise you will not miss these items.

Times Have Changed

The only constant in this world is change—and change is at the very core of the fashion industry. Designers and retailers thrive on convincing us to be consumed with making sure that we have the latest style trend. It can drive you crazy to try to keep up. However, you may be sabotaging your best look by wearing clothes that visually add weight to your frame. Proportion and balance in your clothing is key in accentuating your positive attributes.

Here's an example. I met a new client at a department store to help her shop for updated denim jeans. My client is petite and has concerns about looking shorter. When she arrived, I noticed that the jeans she was wearing were about four inches too long and had fabric bunched up around her ankles. The excess denim visually pulled down her silhouette and made her look shorter. She mentioned most of her pants were too long, and that it was difficult to find something off the rack with the proper length for her. Just by shortening her pants to the proper length, she instantly looked taller and leaner.

It is essential that you find a good tailor or alterations resource. By working with a good tailor, you can transform pieces that do not fit properly. It is rare to purchase something off the rack that offers an excellent fit for any body shape. Critical areas where I see the greatest need for alterations are sleeve, skirt, or pant length. It is worth the small additional investment to get a proper fit.

Finally, almost nothing is more frustrating than reaching for something to wear, only to discover that it needs repair. Don't allow things in need of repair to linger in your closet. Get them repaired right away. Make sure what's in your closet is ready to wear.

Moneymakers

In navigating wardrobe edits, I have found a consistent challenge for many clients when it comes to letting go of things that were a significant investment. Even when an item is the wrong color, silhouette, size, or lifestyle match, if it was expensive, it's hard to let go of. The good news is that there is a thriving industry of consignment shops that will give you the opportunity to get a partial recovery of the money you invested. You will also benefit by becoming familiar with your local consignment shops. As a personal stylist, I am familiar with the kind of merchandise that sells, what various consignment store policies are, and when they accept new merchandise. I coordinate account setup, drop-off, and payment with my clients. It's a great way to earn some cash toward new items that will refresh your wardrobe.

I Remember When . . .

It's fascinating how emotional we are when it comes to our clothing. Often our clothing is tied to a memory or a story. At times these associations are positive and sentimental. Other times memories recalled might be sad but meaningful.

An example from my closet is an old, white sweatshirt that I wore while training for my one and only Team in Training for Leukemia Marathon. During the six-month training program I raised funds for the Leukemia & Lymphoma Society to help support an eight-year-old boy named Joel Green. That sweatshirt represents all the long days and hours of training to prepare for the race. It reminds me that, with commitment and dedication, anything is possible. Anyone who would see it folded in my closet would just think it's an old, frayed sweatshirt. But to me, it's special. Sometimes an item's significance is just too great to let go of, and that's OK. Just store it, and reevaluate during your next edit.

A GIRL'S BEST FRIENDS: ACCESSORIES

So that all your accessories make for memorable looks, when editing the same basic questions need to be asked to determine if you should keep, donate, or consign your items:

- Have you worn it in the last six to twelve months? If not, why?
- Is it in good condition?
- Does it fit your fashion style and lifestyle needs?

- Is it right for your DRES Gem Shape and proportions?
- Is it a good color for your skin tone?

Bottom line: see what accessories you have available before choosing which to wear. The old saying "out of sight, out of mind" rings true when working with your wardrobe accessories.

While working with my clients during an accessory edit, I can't tell you how often great jewelry is rediscovered during our time together. Everything from necklaces, earrings, and rings are hidden away in jewelry boxes somewhere. Here are some great suggestions on how to get your accessories visible in your closet so that you can start enjoying them.

Jewelry

One of my fondest memories from my childhood is playing dress up with my two younger sisters in my grandmother's dresses and fantastic costume jewelry. The dresses were made from incredible, textured fabrics in styles from the 1940s and 1950s. The costume jewelry was bright and colorful, from clip-on earrings to statement broaches. So much joy and creativity came from hours spent putting on our glamorous outfits and then serving each other tea and cookies. Over time the dresses became worn out and my sisters and I moved on to other things, but I still regret that we did not keep all the beautiful pieces of costume jewelry. They weren't heirlooms, but to me and my sisters they were.

I mention this because there is something unique when it comes to jewelry. It is easily stored and will often come right back into fashion years down the road. This is one area for which I suggest a little extra thought be put into each item during your wardrobe edit before you decide to let something go.

Here is what I consider to be the essential list of jewelry for your wardrobe, as a guideline to help with your edit, whether or not you're a jewelry person. Make note of any voids you find, and add them to your shopping list. These core essentials will keep you covered for all those occasions that we will face throughout our lives:

- A set of diamond studs
- A set of pearl studs
- Neutral hoop earrings
- Fun casual earrings
- Dressy dangle earrings
- A diamond pendant necklace
- A statement necklace
- Neutral chain bracelet
- A metal wristwatch
- A simple cocktail ring

Now that you know what is staying in your wardrobe, then decide how best to store your jewelry. One of the most efficient ways is to use a clear vinyl, hanging pocket jewelry organizer. They come in a variety of sizes, and many are two-sided to accommodate different sizes and styles of jewelry. This is ideal for earrings in particular. I also recommend using a canvas necklace and bracelet organizer. These are the best options, particularly when limited on space. Both of these types of organizers can be hung on your wardrobe bar or flat against a wall. For bulkier items, or those that you do not want to hang, I suggest purchasing a few jewelry tray organizers. If you have the space, you can use velvet earring, necklace, and bracelet display fixtures to store and showcase your most commonly used items. This simple change of getting your jewelry where you can see it will make it easy and fun to incorporate it into your daily style. Now is your chance to make a change and use your jewelry to create visual interest and modernize your look.

Shoes

I have yet to meet a woman who doesn't love shoes. There seems to be some inexplicable magnetic attraction between a woman and shoes. Often we will buy shoes without considering the price, practicality, or outfit to wear them with. You just "have to have them." We often go so far as being unconcerned if we can properly walk in them. I'll never forget my first day of freshman year at high school. I wore a pair of the original Candies four-inch high-heeled shoes and hobbled around the halls thinking I looked great. The truth is that I'm lucky I didn't fall or break my ankle. But thirty years later, I still love high heels. I've just had a little more practice walking in them.

Here is what I consider to be the building blocks for a versatile shoe wardrobe. This is a guideline to help you during your edit, not a "must own" list. Your shoe needs are determined by your lifestyle and activities during the week. Climate and culture also play a role in determining your ideal shoes. A perfect example is that here in Texas, you really should have a pair of fantastic cowboy boots. There are a broad range of events where you will need to have those boots for the perfect "Texas chic" outfit. If you live in the northern United States, you will want to have a pair of durable and stylish snow boots. Working with your DRES System Stylist, you can make note of any voids you find and add them to your shopping list based on your specific needs.

- Basic black pumps
- Nude heels
- Metallic gold or silver heels
- Knee-high boots in black or brown
- Flats
- Casual sandals
- Athletic shoes

When editing your shoes, pick a system for storing them that works best with your space limitations. A few options for organizing shoes are:

- A floor shoe rack
- Built-in shelving
- A hanging shoe organizer
- See-through plastic boxes
- Original shoe boxes with photographs stapled to the front, showing their contents

For shoes you don't frequently wear, such as a pair of evening shoes, store them in another area or under the bed. The shoes that you decide not to keep can either be donated or consigned. Don't keep them in your closet creating clutter. It's time to make space for some updated selections. Be sure to keep your shoes in top condition. It's worthwhile to protect your investment.

Having a good shoemaker is as important as finding a good tailor. Most cities will have a good shoemaker. It might take a little research to find them. You can ask for a recommendation from a shoe sales associate at a department store such as Nordstrom. If you are not able to find one locally, I recommend using www.cesarsshoerepair.com out of New York City. For more than thirty years, they have been the leading chain of shoe repair stores there, under the names Andrade Shoe Repair and Cesar's Shoe Repair.

Just a few services a quality shoemaker can provide are:

- Replace half soles and heels
- Replace the shank
- Refinishing uppers
- Replace broken heels
- Replace boot zippers
- Heel lifts
- Leather dyeing
- Apply sole guards
- Add padding
- Stretching
- Professional polishing

The right pair of shoes can make all the difference when it comes to completing a look. Candace Bergen has said that no matter what one's wardrobe costs, if paired with quality shoes, everything looks high quality.

Handbags

Let's be honest: no single bag can meet all your needs. Only a range can cover every aspect of a woman's hectic life today. The goal is to balance what you love with what your lifestyle dictates. Blend a style or color that you love with the functionality that works for your life. Versatility is key.

A basic handbag wardrobe should include:

- A day bag (one for the spring/summer months, another for fall/winter)

- A weekend bag (more casual look and styling)
- An evening bag or clutch

When editing your existing handbags, ask yourself the following additional questions:

- Does it fit the items you carry daily?
- Does it feel comfortable to wear?
- Is it a color that works with most of your wardrobe?

The ideal way to store your handbags is to stuff the inside with paper to maintain the bag's proper shape, and then keep it in a dust bag to protect the exterior. Your handbags should be stored on a shelf and upright, if possible, to help maintain their shape. Just like your clothing, group them by type and style.

Just like clothing, handbags need to be compatible with your DRES Gem Body Shape. Here are a few tips to consider while editing your current bags or for what to purchase based on your body shape:

Diamond: Look for bags that fit into the curve of your waist. If your bag falls too low, it will extend the width of your hip. If your bag sits too high, it will visually extend the width of your chest. Styles that complement a diamond body shape include hobo, messenger, satchel, and envelope.

Ruby: Look for bags that hang to your hip or else carry handbags. If they sit too high, they visually extend the width of your chest. Styles that enhance a Ruby body shape are tote, messenger, satchel, and envelope.

Emerald: Look for bags that hang to your hip or sit high under your arm. If they fall in the middle, they will visually extend your waist area. Styles that enhance an Emerald body shape are tote, messenger, barrel, and satchel.

Sapphire: Look for bags that fit into the curve of your waist or under your arm. If they fall too low, they will visually extend the width of your hip. Avoid handbags that draw attention to your hips and thighs. Styles that enhance a Sapphire body shape include hobo, satchel, barrel, and clutch.

Regardless if it's a statement necklace or a vivid handbag, accessories are a great way to express your creative spirit and adapt trends that fit your lifestyle.

HOW TO ORGANIZE

To have a well-organized and easy-to-shop closet, arrange all your items grouped by category. As you progress with your edit and are making the decisions on what to keep, repair, donate, and so on, the items that are returning because they are "keepers" need to be sorted.

Type and Color

Using the hanging space in your closet, separate your clothing by category, then style, and then color. It's important to hang everything you have room for so that it's easy to see all of your clothing and accessory options. All hangers and items on the hangers need to be facing the same direction.

- Separate your pants, blouses, jackets, suits, dresses, and so on.
- Then organize within the category by style. For example, start your blouses with sleeveless, then short sleeves, then long sleeves.
- Finally, within the category, style sort by color. The color range should go from light hues to dark. I suggest using the following order: white, cream, yellow, orange, red, green, blue, purple, brown, gray, and black.
- Incorporate printed or nonsolid colored items in a group at the end of each category. Follow this same system within every category.

As your closet begins to take shape and you have a visual overview of your items, you will start to discover if you have a tendency to gravitate toward a particular color or style. This is very insightful and a good way to begin to create your wardrobe checklist. An example is from a past wardrobe edit with a client who discovered she had eight to ten ankle-length, casual skirts in a variety of colors and patterns. Previously all of her items (tops, bottoms, jackets, etc.) were mixed together in her closet. By grouping her clothing items, it created an easy way to see her pattern of purchasing the same style of skirt. Not only were these skirts the wrong proportion for her body shape, but they added extra pounds to her look and were clearly an outdated trend.

After having her try on each skirt, we were able to shorten over half of them to the proper length, breathing new life into her wardrobe. My client said it felt like she had purchased five new skirts for only a small alterations fee per skirt. What a great way to stretch her wardrobe dollars and modernize her look! Now when she wants to add to her wardrobe, she knows what style is most complementary to her DRES Gem Shape and how to enhance it. That's a win-win!

THE IMPACT OF YOUR BEST COLORS

Color plays a vital role in how others perceive you and how they react to you. Color is energy! If you're wearing the colors that are right for you, you'll look dynamic. At the same time, if you are wearing colors that detract from your brilliance, there are negative consequences. Everyone has the opportunity to use color in their wardrobe to evoke the response they desire from others. Color is very powerful in changing your look. Wearing colors that flatter you will enhance your best features and instantly make you look more vibrant and youthful.

A common misconception is that everyone should wear black. While working with a client during her edit, her closet was filled with basic black pants, jackets, and skirts. After having her try on a few jackets, I quickly discovered that basic black was not a good choice for her coloring, especially against her face. It deepened the dark area under her eyes, brought out facial lines, and made her cheeks pale and sunken. I determined that a deep charcoal was a much better match.

A good tip that will help during your wardrobe edit to evaluate a color is to look in the mirror and decide what is the first thing you see or notice. If it's not your face, eyes, skin or hair, but rather only the color's boldness, then that color is wearing *you* and you are not wearing the color. The color selection choices in your closet should complement, not overwhelm. Of course, I was not about to ask my client to discard every piece of black clothing in her closet. By being creative with color accents in accessories, we were able to diffuse black's dominant impact and retain pieces from her wardrobe. While evaluating each clothing item during your wardrobe edit, don't discount color. It should be the first consideration on your checklist.

WARDROBE CHECKLIST

Your wardrobe checklist is created from a combination of uncovering your lifestyle needs and activity profile in addition to the missing items revealed in the actual edit. By analyzing your weekly activities and checking off what you already have from the DRES System's core basics wardrobe list, we can compile a list of needed items and then prioritize them according to urgency and available budget.

Wardrobe Core Basics

Regardless of where you live, there are items in your closet that are used year-round. As adults, it's not often that we actually wear out an item in our closet. However, there are times that a frequently worn item gets old and tired looking from fabric weakening, discoloration, piling, or just from normal dry cleaning or washing. Many of these are core basics essential to everyone's wardrobe, no matter your body shape. These are the core building blocks and foundation pieces for creating your individual style. These are also items that typically need to be updated or replaced yearly.

Core Essentials Checklist

SHOES	TOPS	BOTTOMS
1 Pair of Flats	5 Blouses	3 Skirts
1 Pair of Heels	5 Tanks or Shells	2 Dress Slacks
1 Pair of Athletic Shoes	5 T-shirts	1 Pair of Jeans for Heels
1 Pair of Boots	5 Long Sleeves	1 Pair of Jeans for Flats
1 Pair of Sandals	5 Sweaters	2 Casual Pants
		2 Shorts

FORMALWEAR	ACTIVEWEAR	OUTERWEAR
1 Cocktail Evening Dress	5 Workout Tops	2 Light Jackets
2-Piece Suit (Pant or Skirt)	5 Workout Bottoms	1 Casual Winter Coat
		2 Workout Jackets
		2 Swimsuits
		1 Dress Coat—Winter
		1 Dress Coat—Summer

UNDERGARMENTS	SLEEPWEAR	WORKWEAR
1 Strapless Bra	5 Sets of PJs	2 Sets of Work Clothes
1 Push-up Bra	1 Robe	
1 Racerback Bra	1 Pair of Slippers	
14 Panties		
1 Figure Enhancer		
10 Pairs of Dress Socks		
10 Pairs of Sport Socks		
2 Pairs of Solid Tights or Hose		

Once you have a clear and prioritized list, you can begin to use your shopping resources to fill in the missing pieces. Partnering with a DRES System Personal Stylist will ultimately save you time and money. Understand that it can take time to find the perfect pieces to complement your wardrobe. Patience is a virtue, especially when it comes to a fashionable wardrobe. I suggest keeping your wardrobe checklist with you. You never know when you might unexpectedly happen upon a great fashion find.

Here are a few tips from my newsletter, *Monthly Guide to Super Savings,* for when to shop and how to find the best bargains:

- Wednesday is the best day of the week to shop. You will find fewer shoppers, reorganized racks, more sales help, and bigger bargains. Price cuts often happen midweek to get merchandise moving and gone by the weekend.
- January is a great time to buy a special occasion dress. The sale racks are full of them.
- February is the best time to shop for undergarments and bras. Most lingerie companies and stores hold special events and promotions during this month.
- April is one of the best months to shop at your local consignment stores. Women are cleaning out their closets and the consignment stores are filled with new merchandise.
- September is the biggest month to save on denim during the year. The sales are everywhere.

Most women reevaluate their wardrobes in the spring and fall. The process of editing your wardrobe will continually become easier over time. As you become more knowledgeable about your body shape and what brands and fabrics work best, going shopping will no longer be frustrating. Having a well-organized closet full of items that make you look and feel brilliant will be the ultimate reward.

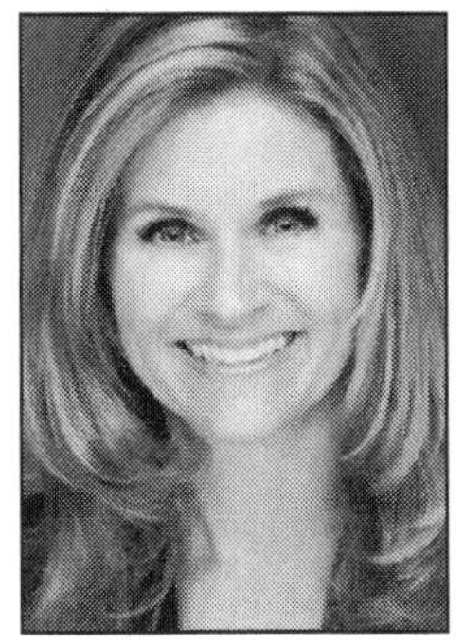

Colleen Bradley

DRES System–Certified Personal Stylist

www.DRESsystem.com/colb
colleen@cbwardrobeconsulting.com
Austin, Texas

Colleen Bradley enjoys helping clients rediscover their signature style and dress with more confidence so that they can consistently feel great.

Before she began as an independent wardrobe consultant using the DRES System, Colleen spent twenty-two years in sales and consulting for a variety of Fortune 500 organizations, such as IBM, E*TRADE, and ADP. Throughout her years of presenting to CEOs, CFOs, and other executive management, she learned to dress smartly without sacrificing individual style.

While acquiring her degree in fashion merchandising, she increased her knowledge of the apparel industry by working for the Dallas Apparel and Accessories Market. This opportunity provided great insight into how your wardrobe and appearance present a strong message to all the people you encounter. Colleen's gift and passion is the ability to use her background in fabric, color, design, and clothing construction to work with clients in translating trends and identifying key pieces for building the perfect wardrobe.

Colleen is a graduate of Texas Woman's University, with a bachelor's in science in fashion merchandising and marketing, and is an alumnus of Alpha Omicron Pi Sorority, Delta Theta Chapter. She volunteers with Dress for Success, a nonprofit organization that promotes the economic independence of disadvantaged women by providing professional attire, a network of support, and the career development tools necessary to help women thrive in work and in life. She is also a dedicated volunteer with the children's ministry at Riverbend Church in Austin. She is married and has a son.

CHAPTER 6

ACCESSORIES

TRANSFORM AND TRANSCEND YOUR STYLE

By Melissa Sabatine

"Accessories are important and becoming more and more important every day. They can completely change the look of an outfit, and women like the idea of having a wardrobe that's versatile. For instance, a strong piece of jewelry can make a simple outfit look elegant."
—Giorgio Armani

As a little girl growing up in Lancaster, Pennsylvania, I never wanted to go anywhere without my sunglasses and handbag. One of my favorite photos from my childhood is of me standing with my mom on our front lawn, a five-year-old diva decked out in my sunglasses and patent leather shoes, earnestly clutching my handbag. When I wore my sunglasses into church on Sundays, our pastor would say, "Here comes the movie star!" At that early age, I instinctively knew that accessories are the universal style booster and how their use could manage others' perceptions. A well-chosen accessory energizes and completes an outfit, personalizes a look, makes a statement, and transcends age.

Throughout my adult life, accessories have continued to reign in my wardrobe. Many a day has passed when a sparkling statement ring or bracelet boosted me through a dreadful work meeting. My handbag wardrobe is so vast that I have opened my closet to a shower of purses tumbling onto my head. I have found accessories to be my best friends after the age of forty, both as camouflage agents and wrinkle reducers. But it wasn't until I became a fashion stylist that I fully began to understand the magical, transformative powers of a well-placed necklace, scarf, or belt, and the confidence boosts the perfect handbag can give a gal.

After receiving some initial training in personal styling, I was in search of a system that resonated with my personal mission: to provide personalized, holistic services. I did not want to simply tell a client what to wear; I wanted to help her feel confident in her total look—from the inside out.

My targeted clientele are those who wish to impact public policy at the federal level. These individuals are playing for high stakes, and it is of the utmost importance that they have a secure sense of personal power. It is critical that they feel confident and project a polished image of authority. These types of clients also like systems. They are too busy and have too much on their minds to have to remember style tips or conversations. They also travel frequently and need to be able to pack quickly and effortlessly. Starting from scratch every time is not an option for them—they need tools.

When conducting some Internet research on various styling systems, on Facebook I came across DRES System and reached out to the founder, Margaret Spencer. She was immediately responsive, and I was fascinated to learn about her art background and the principles on which she created the DRES System. What was most important to me, however, was the warmth and positive energy I heard in Margaret's voice as we chatted on the phone. She really cares about helping others and that was a must-have quality for me in a business partnership.

It also was apparent that Margaret is very passionate about her product and believes in its effectiveness. Many months later, I had the opportunity to meet Margaret in person in Seattle, Washington, and knew definitively that I could stop looking for the best system to build my business. The DRES System is a superior approach with the right tools for stylists and their clients to achieve the best possible results.

I believe that I was led to the DRES System for one simple reason: it is a styling system designed to bring out the inner and outer brilliance in every woman. While the body-shape analysis is a key element of the system, the color and face-shape analyses offer clients a comprehensive suite of services. What women absolutely love about the system is that they are treated like the unique, faceted jewels that they are. In the DRES System accessories are used to reinforce this beauty via the personal style statement created with a DRES System Stylist, and to complement a specific body type and range of colors. As Margaret Spencer notes on her company's website, "We are in the business of confidence."

Introducing new accessories into a client's wardrobe, and teaching her how to use them to enhance her style, is one of my favorite parts of the DRES System's process of creating confidence. By the time I discuss accessories with a client, I have spent a good deal of time with her, gaining insight into her personality, the challenges she faces, and her personal goals. It is exhilarating to help a client choose items that top off her newly found confidence, finding the right color, size, and style for her lifestyle. Accessories can do amazing things for a limited wardrobe budget, and open up new possibilities to tried-and-true wardrobe staples. The perfect handbag, bracelet, or even eyeglasses can also open up newly found confidence—and add a little spring in the step to power through that important meeting, evening out, or public appearance.

ACCESSORIES THROUGHOUT THE DECADES

Looking back over history, the mood of the times and the defining events of every era have been reflected in fashion trends. Taking a journey down memory lane to remember past popular trends can help put some of today's trends in perspective. Indeed, in the spirit of "everything comes back around," you may very well recognize some items that are popular styles today.

1901–1920: The Edwardian Era

The beginning of the twentieth century was a lighthearted time. Fine jewelry projected the mood, with diamonds set in platinum created in intricate lace or garland designs. Shoes, in reality more like elegant boots, were often decorated with bows or fastened with colorful ribbons. Edwardian ladies carried fancy parasols and fans made to match their dresses in designs of silk and lace. The Dorothy bag was very popular at the time, a dainty purse constructed of a square of fabric with a drawstring at the top as a closure. These bags were carried by brides and used as accessories for evening functions. Dorothy bags were often decorated with beads or embroidered embellishments.

1920s: The Roaring Twenties

Women's fashion trends translated the luxuriant and extravagant aura of the Roaring Twenties. Who doesn't love the free-spirited, happy demeanor of a flapper? Fashion accessories such as beaded and sequined headdresses adorned the chic, bobbed flapper hairdo and feather boas. Other notable pieces of the 1920s were long strands of faux pearls popularized by Madame Coco Chanel, plus the adorable cloche hat. In jewelry, the '20s were an age of sparkling art deco pieces. Linear, geometric designs filled the jewelry boxes of ladies of the Roaring Twenties, and those pieces served to lift their spirits in the bleak years of the 1930s.

1930s: The Great Depression and World War I

As the severe economic downturn caused by the stock market crash of 1929 ushered in the Great Depression, ladies' fashion reflected the negative impacts and stresses of the time. Many women turned to filling their closets by making their own clothes and accessories. Conservative, clean lines and understated styles prevailed in women's clothing. Designer Elsa Schiaparelli introduced shoulder pads and the use of a bright pink. (God bless her!) Matching ensembles—think matching a bag with shoes—became more popular, and gloves played very a strong role in wardrobes. World War I and the development of new technologies introduced cheaper fabrics to the market such as the synthetic stocking. And, by the way, that bit of matching shoes to handbags no longer applies!

1940s: World War II

The 1940s are my favorite fashion era—it was a decade that combined style and elegance. Hollywood glamour was at its height with stars like Ava Gardner, Rita Hayworth, and Veronica Lake. Although times were tough, the glamorous starlets gave American women better times and wardrobes of which to dream. Popular accessories of this time included a fire-resistant resin jewelry called Bakelite. Although Bakelite was invented in 1909, it became popular decades later with the availability of pieces in a wide spectrum of colors. Ankle-strap shoes, neck scarves, head scarves, barrettes and hair combs, gloves, and clutches could all be found in the dresser drawers and armoires of 1940s ladies.

1950s: Rock 'n' Roll

The upbeat, new world of rock and roll brought bobby socks and cat's eye eyeglass frames onto the fashion scene. I have photos of my mom in a pair of those beautiful glasses, and I always thought she looked so incredibly chic. Today, those frames are back in style, and I wish she had kept that pair!

I do have something from my grandmother that was popular during this time: a purse with Lucite handles. These clear handles made the fabric body of a purse look chic and sophisticated. My grandma's bag has even another touch that was popular at the time: a mirror in the interior purse pocket.

Neck scarves, saddle shoes, and initials on clothing (like the *L* sported by Laverne in the popular TV comedy *Laverne & Shirley,* from 1976 to 1983) also come to mind when I think of fashion accessory trends of that era.

Another enduring fashion accessory, aviator sunglasses, became popular in the 1950s. After General Douglas MacArthur landed on the beach in the Philippines in World War II sporting these sunglasses, everyone wanted to wear aviators. Ray-Bans became a household name.

1960s: Peace, Love, and The Beatles

The 1960s became known as a time of social revolution. Some historians label the decade as the Swinging Sixties because of the relaxation of social taboos relating to sexism and racism that occurred during this time.

Fashion accessories became an extension of a natural and carefree attitude with flowing scarves, chunky bangles, love beads, and chain belts.

For dressier occasions, ladies opted for pillbox hats popularized by Jackie Kennedy, fur stoles, and elbow-length gloves. Stiletto heels and false eyelashes entered the scene, as did miniskirts. Mod (short for modernist) style became popular with the British invasion of The Beatles and other rhythm and blues or rock and roll bands. These mod ladies often accessorized their looks with patterned tights, feather boas, medallion necklaces, crocheted handbags, and go-go boots.

1970s: The Me Decade

Novelist Tom Wolfe termed the 1970s the "Me Decade," referencing Americans' attitude and their emphasis on the individual during this time. Wolfe cites the economic boom of post-war America as affording the average American a sort of self-determination and individuation.

Women expressed their individualism through nontraditional, decidedly more bohemian clothing ensembles. More traditional belts were replaced with beaded or macramé creations. The use of the skull motif and the peace sign became popular in jewelry, as did the mood ring.

Eyeglasses with very big frames became trendy. The hippie look of the '60s remained strong with the ladies in the 1970s, who did not wish to give up their frayed jeans, go-go boots, and feather boas. The most notable and significant accessory of the decade, however, was the platform shoe. Sporting an average of two- to four-inch soles, platforms came in every design, from solid colors to crazy prints.

1980s: Madonna and *The Official Preppy Handbook*

Personally, this was my least favorite time in the history of fashion and the time of my unattractive high school years. On one end of the spectrum, there was the preppy look made popular by the release of *The Official Preppy Handbook*. Penny loafers, Bermuda bags, and headbands were worn by students all over my high school. On the other end of the fashion spectrum was spandex, leg warmers, and headbands, popularized by the Jane Fonda aerobics rage—and then there was the Madonna factor.

If there is one figure who can be said to have pioneered an iconic '80s look, that would be Madonna. Religious jewelry, rubber bracelets, lace headbands, and armloads of bangles were all on the wish list of every teenage girl. I must admit that I owned a pair of fingerless lace gloves that were a Christmas gift from one of my best friends. They were a beautiful shade of blue, and I thought I was hot stuff when I was wearing those beauties!

1990s: The Information Age

In the 1990s, the United States experienced a long period of economic expansion. Personal income growth jumped dramatically and the digital world began to explode. The World Wide Web was invented, Intel unveiled the Pentium processor, and Hotmail was born. In contrast to the flashier '80s, this decade approached fashion from a more minimalist standpoint. Styles from past decades began to be recycled. Alternative rock and the grunge music of Seattle sound movement made the unkempt look popular. Jelly shoes burst onto the scene along with hair scrunchies and charm bracelets. The wristwatch began to be regarded more as jewelry than as timepiece. Instead of having one watch, ladies began to build watch wardrobes.

2000s: The "Mash-Up"

Most trends in the 2000s came from past decades and included looks like vintage jewelry, aviator sunglasses, and pointed-toe, stiletto boots. Influences from a multitude of developing subcultures, as well as the globalization of cultures in general, brought great diversity to popular style. This diversity was also a newly embraced and acceptable phenomenon, and emphasized that every individual could develop their own unique look.

The increase in celebrities and music artists creating their own brands offered yet another influence to this melting pot of a decade. Among these celebrities were Gwen Stefani and her L.A.M.B. line, featuring bright and dramatic accessories influenced by Guatemalan, Japanese, Indian, and Jamaican cultures, and Nicole Richie's House of Harlow 1960 brand, influenced by bohemian-style accessories.

2010s: ?

What trends will this decade be noted for in fashion's history books? The luxury handbag? Pandora charm bracelets? Statement necklaces? Ceramic watches? Maybe a little bit of all of the above decades combined? Time will tell.

WHY ACCESSORIES ARE IMPORTANT

"Accessories are the true workhorse of any look."
—Nina Garcia

One of my favorite real-life illustrations of the importance of accessories was showcased in the Uniform Project. In 2009 Sheena Matheiken pledged to wear a little black dress for 365 days as an exercise in sustainable fashion. She wore one dress for one year, changing her look with donated and recycled accessories. Using belts, necklaces, collars, shoes, jewelry and more, this innovative fashionista created amazing and innovative looks. Imagine her frustration if accessories had not existed and she had to deal with looking virtually the same each and every day.

In a world without accessories, she never could have made it through a week, let alone a year, without feeling depressed about wearing the same items of clothing every day. Indeed, the Uniform Project would not have been successful without our friends, the accessories.

The marketplace reinforces the significance of accessories in a woman's wardrobe. In 2011, the women's accessories market posted the biggest increase of any fashion business (*Accessories* Magazine, "Census Report," The NPD Group, Inc., 2011).

Increasingly, women are realizing the importance of accessories to communicate their personal style and taste. Accessories are the shinier, sexier sisters to the underpinnings in a woman's wardrobe. They are like the special guest stars on a television show, used to inject excitement, surprise, and interest in the plot that is personal style. Accessories present endless opportunities for outfits, and are the important details a client needs to put the best shine on her shape whether she is a Diamond, Ruby, Emerald or Sapphire.

When shopping or browsing fashion retail sites online, it may be difficult to understand the impact of a single scarf, belt, handbag, or pin when it's sitting by itself on the shelf or in cyberspace. Combined with foundational clothing pieces, though, accessories help create the total look. They are what icing is to the cake and gift wrap is to the present. Accessories matter just as much if not more than the garments themselves, providing an entirely new opportunity for self-expression.

ACCESSORIES: THE HOUDINI IN YOUR CLOSET

As the Uniform Project so vividly illustrates and as I have seen countless times with my clients, accessories are the key transformative elements in any wardrobe. Accessories transform by:

- Highlighting your best assets and minimizing your worst;
- Making last season's outfit this season's look;
- Taking a day look into evening;
- Keeping casual Friday at a professional level;
- Projecting a more youthful or mature image; and
- Turning a bad hair day into a good one.

My favorite jewelry designer Judith Ripka likes to say that her line will take a woman from blue jeans to black tie. A little bit of bling certainly doesn't hurt any time of day! But perhaps the most brilliant transformative powers of accessories are those that take place internally. Confidence, joy, or even a much-needed boost of energy can be stimulated with the right accessory.

Someone I work with had a particularly bad day one week—an injured wrist, a car accident, and other unfortunate incidents. What saved her mood that day was a beautiful new statement necklace she had just purchased. The pop of color and glamorous feel the piece gave her was much needed that day. Who needs therapy as long as there is good jewelry to be had?!

One day, on a particularly long shopping trip with a client at a local mall, we were focused on adding some business basics back into her closet. While an essential undertaking, shopping for basics is not exactly inspirational. In addition, my client was under a lot of stress and particularly tense during this shopping excursion. As we were browsing in one of our last shops, an emerald green leather tote caught her eye, peeking out from a bottom shelf against the wall. My client's eyes lit up as she eagerly seized the bag and immediately flung it on her shoulder with a squeal of joy.

Whether it was the color, the smell of the leather or a combination of factors, her spirits were lifted and she had one of the best weeks at work in a long time. We all deserve to have those items in our wardrobe. A gal just doesn't get that same thrill from a basic black turtleneck.

I also have experienced the power of my own accessories in transforming someone else's mood. A grouchy checker at the supermarket suddenly becomes cheerful and helpful after one of my rings catches her eye. An unusual necklace of mine has started many a conversation at networking events or with a handsome gentleman. My latest fashion finds have been a source of bonding with executive assistants at businesses where I need to quickly set up appointments and phone calls with their principals. It is amazing how a little bling or a fresh handbag can change a mood, get a phone call returned, or open doors!

Some accessory purchases are indeed emotional, although the above example was also blessed by the DRES System Stylist as being consistent with the client's personal style statement. However, strategically adding elements to your wardrobe is an important part of the DRES System.

I feel like a kid in a candy store when I come across great pieces and I can't wait to share them with my clients. My instinct for finding perfect pieces is something I relish, and I always look for items that are multipurpose, thereby stretching the client's budget and maximizing her options. One necklace I chose for a client to wear to a black-tie event, she also wears with a business suit. For that same event, I chose a snakeskin-print Lauren Merkin clutch for her that not only worked that night, but can be tossed in her work tote as a very appropriate hands-free option for day.

An effective way to visually lay out these options is through DRES System's revolutionary and innovative online DRESbook. The DRESbook is a personal styling and shopping service for cataloguing wish list items and creating a living shopping list. By uploading photos, a DRES System Stylist can use the DRESbook to create looks so that clients don't have to worry about what look is best for any occasion. There is even an option to log where, and how many times, an outfit is worn. For busy ladies on the go or who travel frequently, the DRESbook is a must for their styling arsenal.

HARMONIZING ACCESSORIES WITH PERSONAL STYLE

When choosing an outfit's accessories or while on a shopping trip, the most important thing for a woman to ask herself is how the item relates to her personal style statement. The woman who has worked with a DRES System–Certified Stylist will have an understanding of how that statement is reinforced by her body shape and her best color range. An accessory wardrobe must support that statement at all times.

Accessories are a powerful tool in reinforcing your personal brand and creating your own style trademark. Former First Lady and style icon Jackie Kennedy Onassis was known for her signature sunglasses, among many other accessories. Throughout her lifetime, her accessory wardrobe was so distinctive that many pieces were replicated and made available for the retail market.

Coco Chanel strongly believed in the power of pearls to enhance a woman's complexion. She devised a set of three-stranded pearls so that the lower strand could be pulled up and over the upper strand to create a very chic and special look. Jackie Kennedy wore this style of necklace in the adorable and famous photo of John Kennedy Jr. playing with her pearls while she held him in her arms.

Personally, I have reinvented myself several times in my career and worked in many different fields, but my consistent use of accessories has helped to create my image as a fashionista. I am known for my great handbags that I change almost daily, and for seeking out just the right pieces of jewelry for every outfit.

Being known for a signature look has helped set me apart from the rest of the crowd and reinforced my own personal brand. U.S. House of Representatives Democratic Leader Nancy Pelosi wears strands of large pearls. The pearls add femininity but, by being large, also project strength and power, while not causing a distraction during appearances or media interviews. Ann Romney, wife of current presidential candidate Mitt Romney, has become known for favoring a D.C.-based line of bold and artistic jewelry pieces. The pieces not only serve to brighten up her face after countless hours on the campaign trail, but show the voters a lighter side of her personality. Her choice also shows support for an independent designer and small-business owner, a subtle response to her husband's opponents' attacks on her husband's business background and track record.

As a personal stylist and image consultant in our nation's capital, my target clientele is composed of those wishing to make an impact on public policy: politicians, government executives, industry influencers, journalists, and social entrepreneurs. Attributes like confidence, credibility, integrity, and intellect are what they wish to project with their image, and accessories become an important tool in creating an image. Accessories should reflect a client's personality. For example, one of my favorite male lobbyists in Washington, D.C., is known for wearing fashion-forward socks and colorful ties and braces. He constantly appears on the list of most powerful lobbyists because not only is he an out-of-the-box dresser, but also he is an out-of-the-box strategist who gets results. And he looks fabulous doing it!

The right eyeglasses, watch, and handbag all can help to portray a pulled-together, polished look necessary to thrive professionally in a city focused on power and policy. For political candidates and prominent government figures in particular, accessories can become a distraction, especially in front of a television camera. U.S. Secretary of State Hillary Clinton has been criticized for donning an outdated hair scrunchie to keep her hair off her face. Those scrunchies have garnered significant column space while major world events are taking place that are much more worthy of that ink.

Former Republican presidential candidate Michele Bachmann was the subject of a series of news articles in a popular web-based newsletter. The stories focused on whether the pearl necklaces she was wearing during the debates were too large. I just had to laugh. Pearls are the most classic piece of jewelry a woman can wear, yet in the world of politics, opponents will find a way to disparage them.

Subtle, rather than splashy, is the rule of thumb when it comes to life on the campaign trail. I had the opportunity to speak on a panel regarding candidate appearance at an industry conference sponsored *by Campaigns and Elections* Magazine (*C&E*). *C&E* is a nonpartisan publication for political professionals, containing news and other pertinent information on all things related to campaigning. *C&E* also presents several educational conferences a year where it presents the latest trends, information, and training opportunities to political professionals. I was asked to lead a session on candidate appearance for those just getting started in politics, whether they were thinking of running for office themselves or working for a candidate.

It was a very fun session, and I received a lot of interesting questions. Several audience members worked for female politicians and were interested in how to advise the candidates on their campaign wardrobes, especially when campaigning in rural areas.

Two cardinal rules for female politicians are to not dress overly sexy or to appear overdressed. Many of the questions I received after my talk focused on the best ways for candidates with body challenges to look professional and appropriate. The easiest way to accomplish that is with accessories. Scarves and jewelry can be used to help an outfit be appropriately camera-ready and to convey images of authority, competence, and intelligence.

In his book *Power Dressing: First Ladies, Women Politicians & Fashion*, author Robb Young points out that the right pair of eyeglasses can communicate experience and intellect—or be used to downplay an attractive face—when playing in the conservative and serious world of politics. The Kawasaki brand rimless eyeglasses of former Republican presidential nominee Sarah Palin became immediate hot tickets the moment she walked onto the stage at the 2008 Republican National Convention.

Knowing how and when to use (or not use) an accessory is also important when creating the right image. Young also writes about how former U. S. Secretary of State Madeleine Albright always gave her handbag to an assistant so that she could walk into a meeting with her arms swinging like a man.

Accessorizing to project power while still maintaining a feminine edge for a wardrobe is tricky in politics, but it can be done. In 2005, another former Secretary of State, Condoleezza Rice, made headlines when she strode onto a military base wearing a long black coat with gold buttons down the front, which gave it a military feel. The coat blew open to reveal she was wearing tall black boots with high, slender heels. The image projected a confident, powerful woman who was ready to kick butt and take names. If she had worn a boot with a shorter heel, the effect would just not have been the same.

A double standard undoubtedly exists in politics. Women are scrutinized relentlessly for their appearance, while men typically get a free pass. However, men need to pay attention to their look and what they are communicating about their image. Male or female, a candidate has just seconds to make a first impression with an audience. The choice of ties needs to be well thought out, as certain designs can be distracting when captured through the lens of a television camera. Checks and patterns such as houndstooth can create a wavy or moiré effect, hurting viewers' eyes and distracting from a candidate's message. If a male candidate is seated on a stage or other platform at a town hall meeting or debate, not wearing long enough socks will present quite an unattractive look to voters.

"Dress gives one the outward sign from which people can judge the inward state of mind. One they can see; the other they cannot."
—Queen Elizabeth II

To understand the role image plays in politics, we need to note the distinct ways people process information. At a live seminar I attended, the great motivational speaker Tony Robbins said that no candidate can win the presidency unless he or she can appeal to these three ways of learning: visual, auditory, and kinesthetic. The visual person learns by seeing pictures, an auditory individual learns by listening, and those who primarily process information kinesthetically learn by feeling. For example, these voters are interested in a candidate who "feels right" or gives them a good "gut feeling."

Some politicians choose accessories or certain articles of clothing to ensure that their first impression sends a strategic message or brands them in a voter's psyche. For men, the accessory options are limited to eyeglasses or ties. Former U.S. Senator and presidential candidate Paul Simon became known for his bowties and horn-rimmed glasses. It is more common for a male candidate or politician to use specific articles of clothing to reinforce their campaign platforms.

During the 2012 Republican presidential primary race, former Pennsylvania Senator Rick Santorum sported a sweater vest on the campaign trail. Made in America, the goal was to reinforce a message of down-to-earth family man. Since the sweater vest was made in America at a mill in Minnesota, the vest also reinforced a message about putting Americans back to work. The senator also used the vest as a fund-raising promotion—very clever.

Current U.S. Senator Lamar Alexander donned a red and black plaid shirt and walked one thousand miles across the state during his successful campaign for governor of Tennessee in 1978, and wore the shirt again when he ran for president in 1996. He wanted to portray himself as a man of the people, walking among them in what they might wear every day, as opposed to a business suit that would make him look more like a Washington insider.

ACCESSORIZING TO YOUR STRENGTHS

"The interesting thing is people think accessorizing is just for the punctuation of your look, but it can make you look smaller, bigger, fuller, thinner—you can really manipulate your body type with an accessory. It's really shocking."
—June Ambrose, celebrity fashion stylist and author of
Effortless Style: Make Looking Good Look Easy

When shopping for accessories, you will find the most flattering looks by understanding the colors and styles that are best suited for you. To use accessories successfully, it is always better to choose pieces that are in harmony with body shape and height, thereby always drawing attention to your best features. This is another important role of the DRES System Stylist. The DRES Stylist helps her client think outside of the box. For example, there is even a right way to accessorize a winter coat for various body types. Wearing fedora hats will make petite women appear taller, where a vibrant funnel or infinity scarf will add curves to a more slender frame. The total look of any outfit can either support or accentuate a particular body shape, depending on the goal.

EXERCISE? I THOUGHT YOU SAID ACCESSORIZE!

In lieu of a strict workout regimen, there is another option to looking slim and trim! Yes, really! This is not a typo! A polished appearance is achieved through balance, which is why it is so important to have a body shape analysis completed by a DRES System–Certified Stylist.

How a person is put together makes a difference in how that person is perceived. Too many accessories on certain body types can appear flashy, overdone, or inappropriate. Too few can result in an unremarkable look.

Part of being pulled together is by referring back to your DRES Profile analysis and ensuring your accessories are balancing and complementing your body type. Have a slender frame and want to intentionally add bulk? Want to draw attention away from a heavy midsection? No problem. Accessories can add focus to a particular area of your body, highlight your face, and camouflage your tummy.

This is the fun stuff, so let's get started!

MEN ARE LIKE SHOES

Call me a fashion geek if you will, but I love to download fashion-related songs onto my iPhone. Several years ago, singer Shania Twain released a song comparing shoes to men featured on the TV program *Desperate Housewives*. The first chorus makes every woman smile: *"Men are like shoes, made to confuse / Yeah, there's so many of 'em, I don't know which ones to choose."*

We women all love shoes, right? But there are so many choices, it can be overwhelming. Choosing the right pair makes a look come together beautifully. Conversely, the wrong pair of shoes can kill a look. And, although shoes tend to be a comforting purchase when a woman's weight fluctuates, purchasing the right shoes is important when it comes to dressing to flatter a body shape.

For example, women with smaller ankles and calves will look more proportionate wearing shoes with thinner soles and heels, while those with larger ankles and calves achieve balance with more substantial soles and heels. Sapphires should avoid wide ankle straps as they make legs appear shorter and thicker. The clean, sleek lines of classic pumps and ballet flats sans design details can create a slimming and lengthening effect, especially if they are a nude or beige color. A rule of thumb to ensure a flattering, elongating look is to match the shoes to the leg, not the skirt or dress. For example, wear black boots with black tights and nude or taupe pumps with bare legs.

The bottom line is that a lot of factors play into the perfect shoes for the perfect look. A DRES Stylist will help her client find the right choice by evaluating the garments of the outfit, how much leg will be revealed, and the shape of her client's legs—all in concert with body type.

"Cinderella is proof that a great pair of shoes can change your life."
—Unknown

PUT ON YOUR PEARLS, GIRLS!

One year, a dear friend of mine gave me a very special book for my birthday titled *Put On Your Pearls, Girls!* by British accessories designer Lulu Guinness. Known for her whimsical designs and emphasis on individual style, Lulu includes this mantra in her twelve style tips for women. She assigns significance to the letters in *pearls*: Poised, Elegant, Attractive, Radiant, Ladylike, and Sophisticated.

Pearls are essentials and diamonds may be a girl's best friend, but jewelry in general can be the fairy godmother when it comes to dressing your best. More than any other accessory, jewelry acts as a focal point by attracting attention to good points and minimizing figure challenges.

When working with clients who are in the process of losing weight, I like to suggest a great statement necklace to draw up an observer's eye to the client's face instead of to the tummy or hips. The same applies to a great pair of earrings. This is also where the transformative powers of accessories come into play.

Along with the instant mood boost a little sparkle and shine offers, a client will feel taller and slimmer. A piece that draws the eye down, such as a long chain necklace that drapes over the bust, also elongates, especially if worn over a turtleneck. Chunkier, shorter necklaces also draw attention to the bust area. If blessed with slender wrists and hands, a flattering bracelet and a statement ring will accentuate and impress. Chandelier earrings and a collar necklace highlight long, graceful necks. For gals with a smaller bust, large earrings can give the appearance of more volume to the upper body.

Another fun way to wear jewelry is in the hair or on a handbag. The plain black evening clutch suddenly becomes black-tie ready with a sparkling brooch—or that brooch can be used to secure an updo, taking an outfit from work to evening in a flash.

Headbands are a type of hair jewelry, and there are many different, embellished styles on the market. Once reserved for a preppy private-school look and for little girls, headbands can be worn at all ages with a couple of tips in mind. The danger with headbands is that they can make a woman's look seem too young for her true age, but a chic way to avoid that is to pair the headpiece with a low, slick ponytail. Paying attention to a headband's style and material is also important. Little bows or polka dots are not good options, but some rhinestones or beads can look sophisticated and age-appropriate in the right design.

BELT ONE ON

One of my favorite accessory websites is the United Kingdom–based Once Upon a Belt. The site offers a brief history of the belt, helpful videos on how to determine a belt size, how to tie an obi belt, and some fascinating information. A historical rundown notes that for women living in the Middle Ages, the belt was the predecessor to the handbag, as women would carry their purses or their fans on their belts.

First Lady Michelle Obama has helped to illustrate the importance of belts in enhancing a look and defining a figure. She has paired high-end designer belts with pieces from retail stores like J.Crew. Mrs. Obama owns a beautiful collection of waist enhancers, from wraparound belts called obis, to patent-leather ones with ladylike buckles, to skinny embellished belts.

She wears them over sheath dresses and even more formal gowns—a look that is *très* chic. She will be photographed wearing full skirts with a stylish belt, minimizing her hips and accentuating her waist beautifully. The First Lady has learned the style trick that belts are one of the best ways to transform an outfit.

Belts are important tools in a woman's style arsenal, but they can be tricky. The wrong belt can kill an outfit, not to mention your circulation. In recent years, the fashionable belt options have expanded greatly. If you've been intimidated by belts in the past, it is worth taking some time to work with a DRES System Stylist to find the appropriate styles for you.

The style of a belt should depend on your torso length, body shape, and overall height, which means that petite ladies and Emeralds and Rubies look best with a thin low-slung belt. Taller gals or Diamonds and Sapphires may benefit from wider belts. Wearing a belt at the natural waistline helps Sapphires and Diamonds achieve the best look by drawing attention to the narrowest part of their waists.

I have found belts to be the top accessory lacking in a client's wardrobe. It can be difficult to visualize how a belt will add options to a wardrobe, which is why working with a DRES Stylist is a smart idea.

HAUTE HANDBAGS

With the invention of interior trouser pockets in the 1700s, handbags became almost the sole domain of women. Lucky us! One of my favorite birthday cards from a friend reads "Hope you find inner peace. If not, then a killer handbag in the clearance section." Another friend always jokes that a woman should lead with her handbag when she walks into a room.

Suzy Gershman, author of the popular *Born to Shop* city guidebooks, writes in *Best Dressed: The Born to Shop Lady's Secrets for Building a Wardrobe*, "Forget 'you are what you eat.' In public, you are your handbag."

A handbag is often the first thing someone notices when a lady enters a room, which can be either a good or bad thing.

Handbags can make or break a look as they are a tool to add balance and proportion to a look. Choosing the wrong size of bag can be just as bad as choosing the wrong cut or color in clothing. A general rule of thumb is to carry a handbag in a proportion that is the opposite of one's body type. Small- to medium-size bags balance a petite frame while oversized ones are visually more pleasing when carried by tall or curvy gals.

Paying attention to handle lengths is also essential. Sapphires, who carry more weight in the hips, should avoid a heavy bag at the stomach or hip level or they will create more volume in that area. A hobo bag is a very nice choice because it hits under the arm. The same holds true for Rubies, to avoid bulky or chunky bags carried near bust level. A bag with longer straps or a clutch would be more ideal. Plus-sized gals should opt for bags without structure. Slouchy bags won't create additional bulk when carried next to the body.

TO SPLURGE OR NOT TO SPLURGE?

We have all flipped through fashion magazines, our jaws dropping when we see the price tag on a stunning handbag or a pair of shoes that look like they should be featured in the Louvre Museum in Paris. *"How can a pair of shoes cost as much as a mortgage payment?"* we wonder. A Louis Vuitton handbag is reportedly marked up thirteen times its production cost. The Hermès Birkin bag has a waiting list and is produced in limited quantities. Even if a lucky lady is given the opportunity to purchase a Birkin, she must have the means to pay anywhere from $7,000–$65,000, depending on the materials used to construct the bag. And just who is able and willing to pay that price? Plenty of women do, and let's talk about why.

In the world of accessories, there is not much of a middle ground: Quality goes from high to low very rapidly. If we could reach into the magazine and hold those pieces in our hands, we would feel and see hand-stitching, premium leathers, and one-of-a-kind detail. The construction of the Hermès Kelly bag is so complex that a single one can take days to produce. Some design houses have diversified their lines to include more affordable handbags; while those are very nice, they can be offered at a lower price point because they are machine-made on assembly lines and lack the craftsmanship of luxury bags.

Some accessories are forever, some are disposable and trendy, and some are seasonal. Years ago when I was a communications director in the U.S. Senate, the Senate Press Secretaries Association would travel to New York City each year to meet with members of the media. During breaks in our schedule I had one mission: to get to the Salvatore Ferragamo store on Fifth Avenue and purchase a pair of shoes. On a federal government employee's salary, my usual shoe shopping haunts were DSW or T.J.Maxx, but each year I budgeted for a pair of those Ferragamos. I saw those shoes as investments, well-constructed with quality craftsmanship and materials. They are timeless, simply needing new soles as the years pass, and will never go out of style. Items in a classic style are the best investment—definitely worth the splurge and with less chance of buyer's remorse.

Trends, on the other hand, are the opposite of classic. Trends are the new engines of each season driven by color and runway looks. Some fashion industry insiders say that trends begin on the street. With blogging's popularity, some might say trends are born in the blogosphere. However they begin, trendy accessories bring a sense of whimsy to a wardrobe by adding a fresh element with minimal budget impact. Being on trend does not mean one has to break the bank. Enjoying a low price tag means unlimited options in mixing and matching accessories with various outfits. Fashion jewelry is a way to participate in the latest trend craze without a big commitment.

With the sharp rise in the price of precious metals in recent years, the use of mixed alloys has become very popular. Jewelry trade shows like the Vicenza Gold Trade Fair, which occurs winter, spring, and fall in Italy, have been presenting pieces in a bronze alloy that is more pink than brown. The metal is a dead ringer for rose gold but much more affordable. Tiffany & Co.

unveiled such a new metal in February 2012, and other companies like Honora Pearl Jewelry are incorporating pink bronze into their lines.

A lot of what is hyped each season is driven by what is hot with the celebrity market. Indeed, several celebrities have chosen to create their own jewelry lines for this very reason—celebrities' influence sells.

When the HBO series *Sex and the City* was on the air, the hit show drove the fashion jewelry buzz like no other. Women across America were rushing to buy whimsical nameplate necklaces and big flower pins. When the show was made into a movie, famed fashion jewelry designer Kenneth Jay Lane distributed a line of his baubles that were worn by the stars on-screen, as did lead costume designer Patricia Field. Industry magazines such as *Women's Wear Daily* and *Accessories* report on the latest trends, but for the average consumer, it can be overwhelming trying to keep up. Having a DRES System–Certified Stylist in your corner who can track these trends and guide you in the best choices through your DRESbook or StyleGuide offers the benefits without the work. When working with a client, I am already thinking of how accessories can update her wardrobe as we go through her closet. For example, a classic crewneck cashmere sweater could be updated with a lace or embellished collar, or tying on a scarf in the Pantone color of the season makes a traditional leather satchel look current and fresh.

Vintage accessories, which refer to pieces from many decades or eras ago, are another great way to add some inexpensive pop to a wardrobe. With online resources like eBay and Etsy available to anyone who owns a computer, it is easier than ever to acquire vintage. Consignment shops, estate sales, and garage sales still remain great places to find surprise treasures.

My favorite way to wear vintage is to use pieces in my wardrobe that are highly personal or signify an intriguing story. I love that I own some pieces of my grandmother's that can easily be worked into today's fashions. My Nanny, as I called her, is my style icon, and although she is no longer on this earth, wearing her big, colorful, three-strand bead necklace helps me to feel close to her. Her photo sits next to Coco Chanel's on my inspiration wall. Seeing her glorious matching bead and necklace set that I now own always makes me smile and hold my head up a bit higher.

When to Splurge vs. Hold Out for a Bargain

Splurge on:

- Chic, comfortable shoes
- Diamond stud earrings
- Sixteen- or eighteen-inch strand of real pearls
- Fabulous evening bag
- Neutral color leather satchel-style handbag

Look for bargains on:

- Colorful scarves
- Handbags in trendy colors or prints
- Fashion jewelry like acrylic or beaded bangles and bracelets
- Sunglasses

EVERY HALLWAY IS A RUNWAY

It probably is a stretch to say that accessories can rule the world, but I believe it's fair to say that they can rule a wardrobe. The DRES woman is one who knows how to work a room and also knows that every hallway is a runway. She wants to project the best image she can and have fun doing it. The endless possibilities to enhance a woman's wardrobe with accessories sure make it fun to be a girl, but can also be overwhelming. In consultation with a DRES System–Certified Stylist, anyone can learn how to incorporate the right pieces into their wardrobe.

From shoes to handbags to jewelry, accessories can enhance your look, take an outfit from day to evening, and clearly convey a message about a woman's image. Having an accessory wardrobe in your style arsenal will make getting dressed in the morning fast and easy.

Start building an accessory wardrobe with these must-have basics that are trend-proof, foundational, and flexible. Then, add to these items over time in accordance with your DRES Profile:

- Black pumps
- Nude pumps
- White sixteen- or eighteen-inch strand of pearls
- Diamond or cubic zirconium studs
- Black patent-leather skinny belt
- Statement cocktail ring
- Evening clutch
- Double-handled, ladylike satchel
- Cross-body bag
- Sunglasses with UV protection
- A work tote if you work outside the home
- Dressy watch with a leather strap or metal bracelet band

There is one accessory that doesn't require hours of shopping to find, doesn't cost a mortgage payment to acquire, and comes in an adjustable size. That accessory is your smile, the fastest way to transform any look.

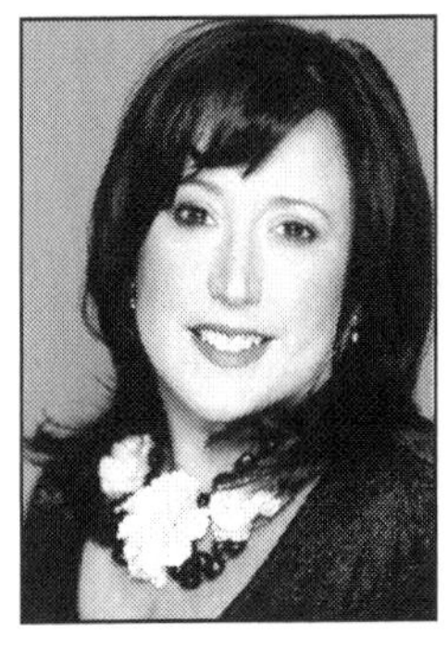

Melissa Sabatine

DRES System–Certified Personal Stylist

Capitol Runway, LLC
www.capitolrunway.com
melissa@capitolrunway.com
Washington, D.C.

Melissa Sabatine is president and chief creative officer of Capitol Runway, LLC, a personal styling and image management service specializing in work with political and public policy professionals and aviation industry executives. Melissa brings over two decades of experience in public policy, strategic communications, image management, branding, and marketing with an extensive network of contacts in both the Washington policy world and the fashion industry.

She serves as the resident fashion stylist for Northern Virginia Fashion Week and is a member of the *Marie Claire* Style Council. Melissa serves on the faculty of The Public Squared, an organization that offers hands-on training for social entrepreneurs ready to engage in public policy. She also serves on the board of the Aero Club of Washington.

While continuing to love being involved in public policy, Melissa longed to find a way to blend her love of that world with her love of personal style and the fashion industry. Those who wish to impact public policy are, in effect, on their own runway, and need to look their best for their message to be communicated successfully. With that goal in mind, she formed Capitol Runway as a one-stop shop, blending her previous political, communications, and policy skills with techniques in personal styling and image management.

Through Capitol Runway, Melissa provides guidance on what to say, how to say it, and what to wear to ensure every client's message is received effectively by someone who has worked in and understands their world.

CHAPTER 7

FACE STYLING

ACCENTUATE THE POSITIVE

By Kat Smith

A wise person once said, "You never get a second chance to make a first impression." I think that's mostly true. I'm sure that on occasion there will be that special person who doesn't judge us on appearance and will not even notice how we look. That person is probably one in a million—or maybe a billion—or maybe that person, like my very sweet, kind Aunt Gwen, is legally blind. So how you look is not her main way of getting to know who you are.

But even without taking looks into consideration, there are many other factors to consider. I asked Aunt Gwen the other day how she forms an impression of someone when she first meets them. She told me that since she has lost her sight, she relies on her intuition and has become very sensitive to a person's energy. She also pays close attention to tone of voice and choice of words.

I have a lovely friend, Chelsie, who is also legally blind. She does have partial sight, so when she first meets someone she takes in the general, overall shape and look of a person. She can see if they are disheveled or put together, how they carry themselves. She just can't see all the details. So she told me that, for her, verbal communication is very important. The words someone uses, the sound of their voice, their tone, if they are nice or rude. When any of us first meets someone, what do we look at first?

For me, it is often a person's hair—that comes from being a hairstylist for a number of years. I can spot a bad cut and color from a mile away! Then the person's face, and then I glance downward quickly to take in the whole look.

Though I work diligently at becoming a more nonjudgmental and enlightened human being, I am not even close to being either. So I do notice how a person looks and how they are put together. And since I am a hairstylist and personal stylist, the visual is huge for me in all things.

Why do I especially focus on the visual? It may be a survival technique. All of us take in a certain amount of data every second. We then take this information and run it through our filters of what we believe to be pretty, attractive, fashionable, trendy, balanced, and so on. How we each go through this process is as individual and unique as we are. We each prioritize which beliefs and filters are the most important for us so, for some, hair is important whereas others just don't care. Some people love or hate tattoos or baggy pants or high heels. The next person may have an over- or underdressed filter with rules around how someone "should" be dressed. And on and on it goes.

MAKING AN IMPRESSION

Much has been written on what it takes to make a great first impression. Who wants to leave a negative impact when they walk away from meeting someone? This is an area in my life where I have experienced struggle and some fear in the past. Because of that I have done research and interviewed friends and colleagues to see what factors are important in making a great first impression. Here are some foolproof steps to take to ensure you create the best impression possible. Remember, you only have seven to seventeen seconds to make those first impressions good ones!

Confidence Is King (or Queen)

Relax; do some deep breathing before your meeting if necessary. Learn how to create the state you want to project. Tony Robbins is a master at this, so check out one of his courses or books on the subject. Don't fidget. A smile is worth a thousand words. Stand up straight and walk with purpose. Make eye contact.

Great Handshake

In my opinion, a handshake says a multitude of things. It shows confidence, power, and self-esteem. When you shake hands, be sure to meet the other person crux to crux, wrap your hand firmly around theirs with all of your fingers, but don't try to hurt them, and step very slightly toward them. That lets them know you are approachable and personable. This is something to practice, practice, practice.

Dress Appropriately

This means "for the occasion." So many times people don't really take into account what they are going to be doing. Do you want to be overdressed or underdressed? What statement do you want to make? Put some thought into the entire look: hair, makeup, accessories, outfit, and shoes. You may be going to a garden party, which may mean wearing a dress and a great hat. What shoes do you wear? Though your five-inch stilettos may look great with your dress, are they going to work walking on the grass? Wedge sandals might be a better choice. And, yes, I'm the voice of experience talking.

Express Yourself

This is just an extension of the above. Your personality should shine through, but appropriately for the occasion. If you're funny, use your humor. If you're not funny but want to be, make sure to practice until you really are funny or you will come across as misguided and will surely make an impression that you did not want to make.

I have a nephew who has always tried to be funny but never really was when he was a kid. He has since worked diligently at it and has crafted a great sense of humor. Like any other skill that we truly want to learn and own, it can be built through dedication and persistence—and practice, practice, practice.

Build Rapport

Know your stuff—about them; if you don't know anything about them, ask them questions. Listen. I will say it again. *Listen!* It is about give-and-take in every conversation. If you talk only about yourself, you are just a bore. Remember the person's name, and use it often. The reason we don't remember other people's names is because we're not really listening.

Follow Up

Whenever you meet someone new, whether for business or as a possible new friend, follow up soon after meeting them. Send a note or e-mail or text just to tell them it was great to meet them—whatever is appropriate for the situation. They will always remember you. This little trick leaves a fabulous impression.

All of this only matters if we want to make a favorable first, or even second, impression on others. We also need to remember that we are never going to be able to leave a great first impression with everyone we meet, as some people are impossible to please. We're not going to worry about them as they can't be pleased, anyway. If we don't care, then it's a moot point. I will assume, though, since you are reading a book about personal styling titled *The Power of DRES* that you do care—and probably care very much how you are perceived in the world. So the question becomes: Why is it important to put my best face forward? Why do I care? It really comes down to the image you want to convey to the world. And is that image the real you or the image that you think the world wants to see? I believe that most people care about their image, their real image. They just don't have the knowledge and tools to make it happen.

YOUR BEAUTIFUL FACE

Face-shape styling is just one chapter in *The Power of DRES*. In my opinion it's tops in importance as your face is at the top of your body and often the first part that we see upon first meeting. In hairstyling we are taught to work mostly with the head shape, using geometry to create all the different looks. (It's kind of funny that the only C I ever got in high school was in geometry.)

In beauty school I was shown how to apply geometry as a creative tool. It was so much more fun to learn it by cutting hair than sitting in math class. No offense, Mr. Lemon! I'm sure you are a great teacher for most. I guess I just needed a fun and creative way to apply it.

I wish more had been taught about face shapes in beauty school, and how important they are to hairstyling and creating an overall look for every client. As I went out into the big, wide world and started my professional hairstylist's career, it didn't take long to recognize how vital it is to know a person's face shape and how it really is the foundation for creating their overall look.

Hairstyle, makeup, and accessorizing: without knowing face shapes and their geometry, we can make serious styling mistakes that will detract from a person's appearance and attractiveness.

POWERFUL ATTRACTION

I have always been curious about what makes someone or something beautiful or attractive. I may be attracted to someone, but my friend just doesn't get it, as they obviously don't see what I see, or don't see the same things the same way. You know, sitting on a bench at a park or at the mall is one of my favorite pastimes. I especially love to watch couples interacting. I have often wondered what they may see in each other because, when I look at them, I may not see what they see at all. Have you ever noticed a couple that looks like they could be siblings, they look so much alike? I know such a couple. I can't wait to see what their children look like.

Have you ever noticed a beautiful woman with a man who is not nearly as physically attractive as she is, and very often he is much, much older? I just assume the man has money. Does that make me shallow? I married for love and attraction, but we all have our own values and priorities.

ATTRACTION'S UNCERTAINTY

I have asked many people the question, "What attracted you to your partner?" There are so many different answers. They say things like, "I fell in love with his smile," or "her eyes," or "I just thought she was so beautiful."

Then I ask, "What is it about her that is so beautiful?" Many times when I ask this question, I get the "Everything about her is just perfect . . . beautiful . . . pretty." They are unable to be very specific because they just see the whole package that they are attracted to. So I did a little research about what makes us more or less attractive to others. Some of the factors that make someone attractive to us are their smell, the sound of their voice, facial features, perceived financial stability . . . and kissing. I love all of these, especially the kissing! There's also a scientific formula called the golden ratio, or the golden proportion. It explains what makes a person's face more beautiful and attractive.

HOW IT ALL STARTED

Margaret Spencer, president of Holobi, LLC, and creator and founder of the DRES System, teaches about the golden ratio in the proportion chapter of her training program. It is a mathematical formula used to determine attractiveness or beauty. The short description is that a perfect face is two-thirds as wide as it is long. How many of us are perfectly equal or symmetrical? Not many, but apparently Brad Pitt fits the ratio perfectly.

Well, of course he does! It is really just a general way to begin studying how a person's face looks.

It tells us that the more a person's face shape fits into the parameters of the golden ratio, the more attractive they will appear to be. Many studies have been conducted that ask the question: "Is there a way to measure attractiveness?" It has been thought that symmetry and perfect balance in facial features is the key. Apparently, though, this isn't the case.

"Symmetry only accounts for 10 to 20 percent of the attractiveness rating. There are other factors that come into account: youthfulness, how feminine or masculine your face looks and how childlike, soft or round your features are" (Mounir Bashour, MD). Thus the attraction to cute babies' faces.

Have you ever seen someone who you think is attractive but in an unusual way? Or do you have friends who are attracted to a certain type of person, but it's a type that you are not attracted to, at all? I have a friend who is always attracted to nerdy-looking men with big noses. Don't laugh! Honestly, that is what she likes. I am more attracted to a rugged-looking man who has some facial hair. Men who are too perfect-looking or too pretty do not attract me. I have known several people who notice teeth as the very first measurement of attractiveness. If the person doesn't have teeth that meet some preconceived expectation, they are out. So there are exceptions to every rule, but the golden ratio is the standard for beauty and attractiveness.

POWERFUL FACE SHAPES

There has been much written about face shapes, just as there has been about body shapes. The descriptions are usually round, triangular, rectangular, oval, long, apple-shaped, or pear-shaped. Personally, I don't want to be any of those shapes. None of them sound very fun or pretty. I love the DRES System's gemstone definitions of face shapes—they sound much more glamorous.

Since I have always been fascinated with what makes a person beautiful, I realize how a woman wears her hair and makeup can change how she looks to express who she is, or who she wants to be. The most important fact that attracted me to the DRES System is how it breaks this all down into an understandable concept that can be used to every woman's advantage.

We each have a precious gem body and face shape, so we each have two gem shapes. Our face and body shapes can be the same or different. How great is that? I personally have the same face and body shape. (I'm an Emerald.) The DRES System gives me the skills and tools to enhance my body and face shape so that I always look my best, just as it will for you.

With the DRES System's mathematical formula, we can determine which precious gem of a face shape you have. The gem shapes for the face are the same as for the body; this keeps it consistent and simple to remember. The four face shapes are:

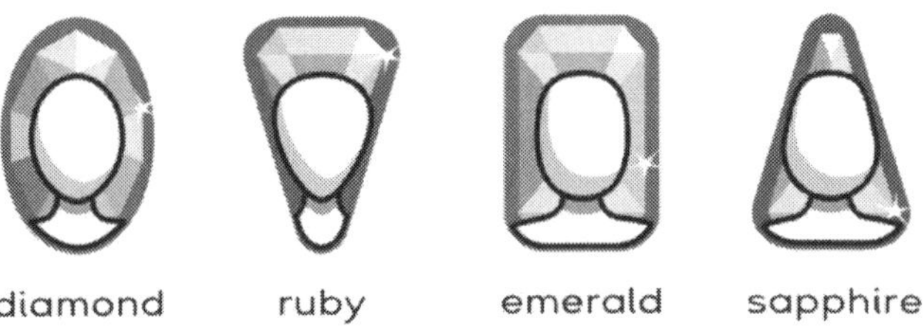

Diamond: The diamond is considered the perfect face shape. It most exemplifies the golden ratio concept. The diamond shape has similar forehead and cheekbones with a narrower jawline. A diamond face shape can wear practically any hairstyle.

Ruby: The ruby-shaped face has a wider forehead than the cheekbones with a narrower jawline.

Emerald: The emerald face shape has similar forehead, cheekbones, and jawline width.

Sapphire: The sapphire has a narrower forehead than cheekbones with a wider jawline. The goal is to slightly widen the forehead.

THE LONG AND THE SHORT OF IT

There are also different variations within each face shape. For instance, a person might be an Emerald, but her face is also very short (my face shape). Another Emerald might have a long variation, which would look a little more like a rectangle. So for every face shape, there will be a long, medium, or short variation. And with each variation, there is a way to create more balance and symmetry.

Let's take my short Emerald shape as an example. I don't want to create too much width at the sides of my face or it will make my face look even wider. If I wear my hair a little longer than my chin and pretty straight, it will make my face look a little longer. I really look my best with my hair short, with some height on the top to slightly elongate my face, and short at the sides to narrow it just a bit. I should not wear a full bang, either. A full bang would close off my entire forehead and make my face look even shorter.

Once we know what our face shape is and whether that shape is long, medium, or short, we can move on to the really fun part. So if the goal is to create more balance and beauty in the face and overall look, we need to go back and look at the golden ratio. This mathematical formula gives us what we need to create our best look. We can then study all of the individual parts of our face and see how those parts look in relation to our whole face. As we look at each part of our face in greater detail, we can ask:

- How far apart are our eyebrows, and are our eyebrows even?
- Are our eyes evenly spaced or are they set wide, or very close together?
- Are our eyes smaller or larger?
- Are our lips full or thin, or somewhere in between?

You get the idea. It's all about balance and proportion. This is not a place where we are allowed to become critical of ourselves, either. No one is perfect and there is no such thing as perfection. We have all seen a model or movie star or two who *looks* perfect, but photographs of these women are often airbrushed—as the women themselves often are, with makeup! If we met them in person, they may not look quite as perfect. If they are that perfect, congratulations to them! They have been super blessed by a spectacular gene pool.

I have met a few women in my lifetime who, I think, fall into this category, but even they seem to have some aspect they don't like about themselves. Sometimes that one thing is what really sets them apart. I have a friend who had a slight overlap on her two front teeth. I just thought it was a beautiful and unique part of her, and I loved her beautiful smile. But she always hated it. So as an adult she had braces put on to correct the problem. Her teeth are now perfectly straight. She loves it and feels much better about herself. Though I think her teeth are gorgeous, I still miss the smile she had when I met her. It was something that set her apart and was unique to her. By looking at someone's teeth, it is easy to know that they have had braces. Really, "perfect" does not always mean interesting.

Hollywood is the spot to see this in so many forms. You'll watch a film with an actor or actress whose looks you like just as they are, and then a few years or movies later, they look so very different, you don't even recognize them! They have had that much "work" done.

An example of this is the actress Jennifer Grey. She had surgery to change the shape of her nose. Did her nose look more perfect? Yes. Did she look like herself? No. Did she look better or worse? That is up for debate. She is one of my favorites, so I don't care what her nose looks like. I just want her to continue acting, so I can enjoy watching her movies.

This is not my meaning when I write about creating balance. The point is not to look like someone else—it is to look like your best *you*. It just requires a few more tools to then take what you have and make it shine, naturally.

THE OBJECTIVES FOR EVERY FACE SHAPE

Diamond: The only variation here is length. So the goal would be to either lengthen or shorten the face.

Ruby: Since the ruby face shape is wider at the forehead, the trick for balance is to widen the cheek and/or chin area. Do this to degrees depending on how long or short the face.

Emerald: This face shape can be fairly square, so the idea is to soften the edges of the square and create length if the face is short or shorten it up if the face is long.

Sapphire: The sapphire shape is wider at the jawline, so the point here is to create width in the forehead.

POWER CONSULTATION

Where do most of us go for our beauty advice? The salon, of course. Going to the salon should be a fun and exciting experience, though, as you may have also experienced, it can sometimes be a disaster. So much of it depends on the communication that happens between you and your hairstylist during the consultation process. Being a stylist for many years means I have done many, many consultations, and by "many" I mean thousands. Every hairdresser has his or her own style and process for a consultation. So here are some stylist evaluation questions for the *okay, better,* and *best* consultation.

Okay Questions

- Do you have a picture of the style you want?
- Do you want to look at some books to find a style?
- Do you just want a trim?
- Are we going to do what we usually do?

I'm sorry to say that that can be the extent of the conversation. Sad but true. Short but not so sweet.

Better Questions

Here is a much better version of the salon consultation:

- Did you bring a picture with you of the style you're looking for?
- (If not) Do you want to look at some of our style books?

It's important to note that the same questions are asked again but with several follow-up questions. A picture is very helpful for the stylist, as stylists are very visual and a picture can speak louder than words for them. With picture in hand, then, another discussion should start with these:

Best Questions

- What do you like about it?
- Is it the overall shape, color, with bangs or lack of bangs, length, or did you like the whole look?
- What's the main reason you chose this particular picture?

Sometimes this was helpful to me, and sometimes the client would just have a blank, bewildered look. Often the answer to all of the above is "I just think she is so pretty, I want to look like her."

People don't often take into account whether they have similar hair texture, thickness, waviness, or straightness in their own hair. That is the job for the hairstylist to determine. Is the picture realistic for the client? Is it possible to achieve the look with what the client has to work with? The sad part is that I have seen so many stylists just take a look at the picture and start cutting, and even though they may cut the same shape in the hair as in the picture, it may not look right on the client. They may have ignored too many of the important factors it will take to create this overall look. It is my job to help them figure out exactly what it will take to achieve the look they desire, if it will be a good look for them, and if it is even possible. If they are a returning client, there may already be a plan in place, so that would be the topic of conversation. The stylist would make sure that the plan was still the same or if there are any tweaks or changes that need to be discussed. And then I continue through the procedure I discussed earlier.

Here is where more questions need to be asked about how they style their hair now:

- How much time are you spending now on your hair every day?
- How much time are you willing to spend?
- What tools do you currently use?
- What tools are you willing to learn to use?
- What products are you currently using?
- Do you like product in your hair or do you like a more natural feel?

By this time a client is often looking at me like I have three heads. Then there are clients who come in and say, "Just fix it. I don't know what to do with it. Just make me pretty."

Those can be dream clients—or they can turn out to be the clients from hell. If I were to just do something without having the information from my typical questions, I could create a huge disaster. Have you ever just said "I want to try something new," and left the salon with some asymmetrical new style the hairdresser just learned about at the last hair show they attended and were just dying to try, and you walked in on the perfect day? You got the new do, and you hate it. You're not sure what's wrong with it, but you know you can't possibly go out in public looking like this. And who gets blamed? That's right, the hairstylist, though both of you share responsibility for the calamity.

Communication. It must come from both positions of the chair in this partnership. It's never enough to say, "I want something new," and just leave it at that. There has to be a discussion between client and stylist on specific likes and dislikes and what outcome is both desired and achievable.

POWER CONSULTATION WITH A FACE SHAPE–CERTIFIED STYLIST

When you don't get what you want from a consultation at your hair styling salon, the problem comes down to two things: communication with the stylist versus advanced consultation tools and skills. Many stylists just don't have the training to do an advanced consultation. They take haircutting and coloring classes, but don't learn how to expand their consultation toolbox.

The questions asked in the *okay* and *better* sections above are a great start, but still don't get you the most thorough consultation possible. We have left out the most important component in the equation: face shape.

I'm curious how many salon stylists take clients' face shapes into account. From my research and in talking with salon owners, it seems to be a thing of the past and isn't taught in any depth by beauty schools any longer. I'm personally shocked and saddened by this. Knowing a person's face shape is critical to giving them their best look. It is the foundation for all haircut and makeup creations.

I was taught a little about face shape in beauty school. It was just the basics, but I took that knowledge to the salon. When a new client would come in, I would give her face a quick once-over and come up with what I thought was her face shape. I had no real way of determining the exact shape, only my best visual guess. It took years of experience to hone that skill, and I always wished there was a way to be more exact in determining a client's face shape. With the DRES System's face shape mathematical formula, I was finally able to do just that. Now that I can pinpoint any client's face shape, and the long and short within that shape, it helps me to figure out where to add or decrease volume, or where more or less length is needed—all of the essential information to give clients their best possible overall look overall. A look that is the most flattering and appealing for every one of my clients. Now I have more, and less, options to style their hair and virtually no room for error with their overall hairstyle shape. I have now given them the most comprehensive advanced consultation possible.

THE NEXT LEVEL

Let's talk about going to the next consultation level: facial features. Once I know your face shape, I'm able to look further to study your individual facial features.

How does each facial feature—nose, eyes, eyebrows, mouth—relate to the other? How does it relate to the golden ratio? If you recall, the golden ratio works to create balance, and not perfection. I am not suggesting a cookie-cutter, one-size-fits-all hairstyle. Each person is unique.

In working with your hair, every good hairstylist wants you to look like the best *you*—that usually just takes a few little adjustments with makeup and hair. Not everyone needs a full makeover, though that is a really fun thing to do for yourself every once in a while. Change is good and healthy, and we all experience times in our lives when we want to or even feel that we need to make a really big update to our look. It may be that we are looking to earn a promotion at work or make a career change, have a milestone birthday coming up, or perhaps it's simply time for a change. The best part is that, as a professional personal stylist and hairstylist trained in the DRES System, I have a precise scientific process to look at each facial feature individually, and then overall, to make adjustments so that your features harmonize well together. I have the tools to design your best overall look.

This might involve hair coloring and a new cut to perfectly enhance your facial shape, features, and skin tone. Your makeup would become flawless, and you would learn exactly what colors and shades to use to balance and enhance your features. In the future, then, when you prepare for your day, you will know what shapes, sizes, and colors of accessories are your most flattering choices. You'll also know flattering techniques for makeup use, how to best wear scarves, and the ultimate colors to light up your life.

THE POWER OF FACE SHAPE

So let's get to some specific face shapes and scenarios and what this process can really do for you.

Bangs

First, let's talk about hairstyles, and bangs, in particular. Here are a couple of scenarios to give you an idea about what a good hairstyle can accomplish.

While watching the televised Miss USA Pageant the other night, I was intently studying the contestants' face shapes and how they wore their hair. All of them had long hair, but it was interesting to see who wore bangs: not many. One contestant I noticed had a Ruby face shape, so her forehead was wider than her cheeks, and she had a small jawline. She had created some fullness at her jawline, which was good, but she had no bangs. She had a perfect face shape to wear a partial, side-swept bang. This would have narrowed the width of her forehead and created more balance with her jawline.

I studied another contestant who wore her hair long and very sleek and straight. Her face was rather long as well. This wouldn't normally have been a great look for her, but she wore full, heavy bangs across her entire forehead. This was brilliant! It shortened the length of her face to a better ratio. She looked absolutely amazing with those bangs. So striking.

Hairstyling

Don't: Have you ever seen someone with a long rectangular face who wears a short, spiky haircut? I normally see more men wearing this hairstyle than women. All that height on top of the head with no hair on the sides just makes an already long face look even longer.

Do: I love a well-done, bob haircut—especially when it surrounds a square face. A proper bob needs to be longer than chin length if the face is short, but nothing rounds out a square face quite like a softly rounded bob. It softens all the corners, nearing perfection!

Eyeglasses

Picking out your own eyeglasses can be very challenging and a bit overwhelming. But don't stress. Here are a couple of examples to get your creative juices flowing.

I have a friend who has a very square face. Her face is also very angular, and her features are what are often called chiseled because she is a professional bodybuilder. She has almost no body fat—she's all muscle. If she didn't choose her eyeglass frames carefully, she could make those angles even sharper, especially if she chose square-shaped eyewear. The best shape eyeglasses for her would be something curvy or round, like aviator-style frames.

So the opposite is true for someone who has a very round, soft face. This person can wear glasses with a more angular or rectangular shape, and give a rounder face a little more definition.

Makeup

An important trick here is knowing how to elongate a short face and shorten a long face. We do this by contouring. To elongate a short face, use a slightly darker foundation or powder shade on the sides of your face; then use the same color at each corner to make a slightly rounded appearance. To shorten a long face, use the same idea but apply the darker foundation or powder across the forehead and chin to create a slightly wider look.

You only have to look at the color of your eyes to find the best eye color and shadow shades. Go for contrasting colors, not necessarily complementary shades. This will make your eyes vivid and memorable.

ACCESSORIZING THE FACE

We certainly don't want to forget this. I find it amazing what accessories can do to completely pull a look together. I'm thinking scarves, necklaces, earrings, and bracelets. This is my favorite part about getting dressed because it's a great time to really be creative. One of the most important things to remember about accessorizing is editing. Put on everything you want to wear, take a look in the mirror, and then remove at least one accessory. Yes, it's what I do so that I don't end up looking like a Christmas tree. Coco Chanel said it best, *"Before you leave the house, look in the mirror and remove one accessory."*

When wearing earrings, a necklace, bracelets, and possibly a scarf, too, make one of those things the focal point. So if you wish to wear a large, chunky necklace, wear smaller earrings that don't make as much of a statement. See where I'm going here? Choose one piece as your focal point and the rest of your pieces to accent or complement—not compete. It's not necessary to wear a ring on every finger just because you can. It would be hard to notice any when there are many.

If you have a longish neck, wear longer earrings. Women with short necks have a harder time wearing those long, beautiful chandelier earrings as they tend to lie on our collarbones—not exactly how they are supposed to look. We just need to find smaller chandeliers.

Longer necklaces will elongate the face and neckline, though they may not always be appropriate with every outfit.

My hope is that the salon of the future will have trained all of their staff in the DRES System's face-shape styling techniques and even keep a few DRES System Personal Stylists on staff to take care of every client's entire look, from head to toe. What would this be like?

Step One: When calling a salon, it would be for an appointment for a DRES System face-shape consultation.

Step Two: After your consultation, your hairstylist, personal stylist, or makeup artist would talk with you about their personal recommendations for your look. This process would take about forty minutes.

Step Three: You would have the chance to go over all your information discovered in your consultation and decide which services are your top priorities. Or you could also possibly make an entire "Best Look" plan with all the steps it takes to get you there. It might be a new cut and color, brow shaping, learning new makeup techniques, a new skin-care process, a personal styling appointment to find your Gem Body Shape, personal styling consult, forty-two Ultimate Colors analysis, closet edit and organize sessions, and more. One-stop styling would all be in one place, and you could have your own entire team of beauty and image experts to help you be the best you can possibly be!

The good news is that we are currently bringing the DRES System Stylist and Face Shape training to salons. This would mean that very soon you could get this full and comprehensive program at your favorite salon. Here is what your salon could provide:

Advanced Face-Shape Consultation: After this appointment you would come away with a fully mapped-out plan for your hair color and style, makeup tips to best flatter your face, best accessories suggestions, and even ideas for your best eyeglass shape.

DRES System Profile: With this consult, you would discover your body shape, fashion style, color range, and more.

Organize and Shop Your Closet: Your stylist takes the information gathered from your DRES Profile appointment and then edits your closet to discover what clothing already works plus what items you need to create a perfectly well-rounded wardrobe.

Personal Shopping Appointment: A trained stylist takes you shopping to fill in the blanks to create that well-rounded wardrobe.

Color Analysis: A personalized analysis using five hundred color swatches to find and give you your forty-two Ultimate Colors Palette. This tool will not only help with wardrobe purchases but will also give you the needed tools to make the best hair color, makeup, and accessories choices. You will always know exactly which colors are the most complementary for your skin tone.

IS YOUR HAIRSTYLIST DRES SYSTEM–CERTIFIED?

It's really all about having more tools in your "best look" beauty toolbox. The more tools, the more options. Experiencing the DRES System's face-shape consultation provides the knowledge you need to make *your* best choices in hairstyle and color, makeup shades, and their application techniques. No more trying a hundred different haircuts over time that never look quite right, then waiting months for them to grow out only to try something else again. No more spending hundreds of dollars for makeup that isn't the right shade.

You will know what works for you and what doesn't work—and why. Changing your look becomes easy and fun because you know you will no longer make the mistakes of the past.

Now, go out and live your best life and look fabulous doing it!

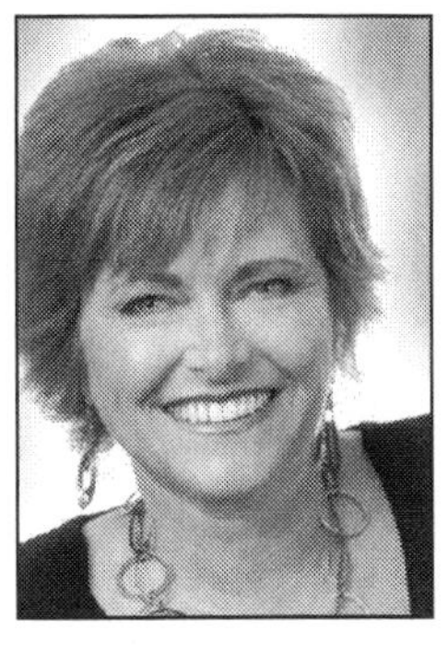

Kat Smith

DRES System–Certified Personal Stylist

www.DRESsystem.com/kats
meaningfuljourney@gmail.com
Portland, Oregon

Kat has always been a fashion and beauty maven. As a preteen, her mom taught her to sew. She spent many hours poring over fashion magazines to see what the trends were; then she would head to the fabric store to find a pattern and fabric to make her own version of the current trends. She didn't just want to be hip and fashionable, she wanted to be fashion-forward. Just the act of getting dressed every day has always been an exciting and creative adventure for her. As her mama says, "Every day is a costume party!"

Hairstyling was another passion of hers. She took cosmetology training in her early twenties and spent many years as a hairdresser and then as a salon owner, specializing in color and stylist training. At Redken on Fifth Avenue in New York City, she learned advanced cutting and coloring techniques. During these years she adopted the hairdresser's wardrobe: black, black, and more black.

After selling her salon and scaling down her clientele, she looked for other creative outlets. She found it in painting: canvas, walls, you name it. She became addicted to color. Her passion for color and fashion were once again ignited. She had once again found her mojo!

Throughout her life, Kat has been passionate about personal growth. A self-proclaimed self-help junkie, she has read and studied many different philosophies, religions, and self-help gurus' teachings. Her life reflects a calm, steady flow that attests to the inner work she has done through the years. She has been happily married for thirty years. She and her husband have two little barky dogs they adore. They split their time between Vancouver, Washington, and Phoenix, Arizona.

CHAPTER 8

MAKEUP

MAGIC AND MYSTERY

By Brenda Azevedo

We have all seen that woman who seems to own her power. Her clothes, her makeup, are perfect regardless of what life throws her way. Was she a little girl sitting at her mother's knee watching and learning all the ins and outs of makeup and style? Or was she a tomboy, without benefit of advice from a stylish mentor? Do you know the roots of your makeup beliefs? Who or what helped to create the pages of your internal beauty book?

I grew up with a mother who did not have the slightest interest in the aesthetics of womanhood. I never heard "you need a slip with that" or "always wash your face before heading off to bed."

If you needed a vacuum or toaster repaired, however, my mom was your gal. As you can imagine, I grew up not knowing a thing about hair, clothes, or makeup. I navigated my way through my twenties with some beauty looks that make me cringe now as I look at old photos.

GIRLS JUST WANT TO HAVE FUN

I must admit I was most comfortable in the 1980s when everyone around me was wearing the same sort of style *costume*. I felt for the first time that I was in step with the masses. For that period of time, I fit in without much effort on my part.

Many of my current clients laugh about the looks of the '80s, but I find if there is a makeup faux pas they committed, it has its basis in that decade. Big hair, big shoulders, and strong eyes topped off with strong lips, oh my! As fate would have it, I ended up in, of all places, the beauty business, when an injury caused me to make a sudden career change. I became the very unstylish owner of a very successful day spa.

I worked hard in the background to allow women to forget their cares and indulge in relaxing treatments that fed their souls. Then a funny thing happened: once my spa clients were relaxed and present in the moment, they looked up and really looked at me. What they saw made many of them want to take me on as a "project." It was agreed that my outside did not match the successful businesswoman they knew me to be. Luckily, for me no one held back. The prescription? It was off to see a stylist for me. I was to have my colors, makeup, and body analysis done ASAP.

THE STYLE DOCTOR WILL SEE YOU NOW

The stylist I was scheduled to see was well known in our local area for her transforming skills. The big day finally arrived, and I was forced to come face-to-face with my outer self for the first time. I had to look at my eyes, my hair, the shape of my body and how it all worked (or didn't work). I had to look at how I was showing up to the world. It was uncomfortable and freeing at the same time.

Old beliefs from childhood were everywhere, on my face and in my clothing choices. I never considered that I was short in stature or that my long, flowing dress was making me look even shorter. None of my makeup, hairstyle, or clothing choices took into consideration any part of the real me when I had made those choices. My goal was to be presentable, comfortable, and to not be noticed. Sadly, I was successful in the not-being-noticed part. I was a businesswoman, but my look was not reflecting that to the world.

With certainty I can say that one day changed me completely. It was not an easy process for me to look at myself critically. It did take me some time to implement all the new style information I was taught and to integrate it into my daily life. I was fascinated how firmly my brain held onto the old picture of me, refusing to really see what was right there in the mirror. I was in my childhood style groove, the comfortable place of old tried-and-true beliefs like, "Oh, I don't wear this or that," or "Makeup is time consuming and difficult." I had to stretch myself. What I learned through that process, and I do know for certain, is that my outdated picture that lived in my head isn't unique. If I was seeing myself incorrectly, could you be, too?

Working in the makeup and style areas of the beauty business, particularly with the DRES System, has been enlightening. I see hundreds of women, so I hear and see many of the same makeup issues. I'm going to condense some of the most common makeup don'ts (names have been changed to protect the guilty) and share some of my clients' makeup stories with you. See if you recognize any of your childhood or early makeup beliefs that may not be serving you now.

Laura Lips

Laura watched, fascinated, as her mother applied her lipstick: how her mother carefully blotted with tissue, looked two or three times in the mirror, correcting and perfecting her lips before she headed out the door. In fact, Laura Lips can still hear her mother's makeup advice in her head: "Never leave home without your lipstick on." Laura could watch her mother for hours, mesmerized by the ritual.

As Laura grew into an adult, she has been continually on the hunt for the perfect lip color. She is drawn to dark lip liner and that, oh, so pretty, bright-coral lip color with extra shimmer that her mother wore. To this day, Laura never leaves home without that jarring color adorning her lips.

Well into her fifties now, Laura is striking and has taken great care with her health and her body. She is fit and fabulous. Sadly, Laura's lip choice destroys any ability to see her as youthful. That dark lip liner and garish lip color age her and command everyone's full attention. You can't see past it! A lesson for all of us to remember: if you outline your lips with a dark color and choose unflattering lipstick colors, it's as if you put a harsh, neon underline through a beautiful picture.

Connie Cosmetic

As a teen, Connie loved getting together with friends for sleepovers. Seemingly every weekend, the girls would spend the night at one house or another, trying on all the new products they found in the pages of *Seventeen* Magazine. All the girls admired Connie; it seemed she was a natural at applying and wearing makeup. Connie went from au naturel to a bronzed beauty in about ten minutes. Connie just loves the healthy orange undertone her powder gives her. Connie's complexion was so "perfected," it almost looked like she wore a mask that could be taken off and on as she wished. Her girlfriends were in awe.

To this day, Connie feels comfortable and competent in her makeup application. In fact when she has had her makeup professionally applied, she is never happy. In spite of raves from her friends and family, Connie feels the makeup artist is always lacking skill. The makeup artist always makes her look pale and pasty. Connie quickly applies bronzer to recover her orange glow and, oh yes, only half the time will she remember to blend it down her jawline. The sad reality is that trying to capture a bronzed glow with foundation is very aging. The darker shade will create shadows and accentuate any fine facial lines, not to mention that orange may not be your color!

Nancy Natural

"Nancy Natural" rounds out our last example. Nancy is a serious student and has excelled in all her scholastic pursuits. Primping was frowned upon in Nancy's home and looked on as representing frivolous behavior. All through high school, Nancy was able to dodge using any mascara, gloss, or powder. Nancy's inner voice has always whispered to her that she must avoid the pursuit of style and makeup as she must be taken seriously.

Now that she is aging, Nancy has wanted to explore using makeup and to learn more about her personal style. Nancy's skin has changed quite a bit and has some red blotches she'd like to cover. Coworkers are commenting that Nancy is looking tired. As Nancy considers her makeup options, she feels fearful—her inner critic continues to play the old, negative, "don't be vain" self-talk tape.

Nancy has been in a makeup holding pattern for years, stopped somewhere between nothing or what she thinks is her only makeup option: to be overly made up. She is not aware that she could be enjoying the benefits and the beauty of a natural, appropriate, and polished makeup application. Choosing to do nothing, Nancy has started to feel like a failure. It's just all too hard.

I know I have been blessed in my life and my business to have come into contact with many different women. Women share and teach freely. Many of my most important lessons have come by way of identifying within myself what other women have struggled with.

Once you discover and embrace your own signature style, you can streamline your routine. The statement "it takes a village" can be applied to many different aspects of life. Well, it really does. Hire that style expert! She will give you the tools and focus to help you communicate to the world who you really are. With a beauty road map it can be effortless. I know that it is easy to discount our outward appearance. I hear "I'm too busy," "it's not important," or "it's expensive." Beauty *is* from the inside out, after all—we all know that. But the truth is, when you are comfortable in your own skin, you feel better about yourself, and you are able to take on the world in a more powerful way.

"Create your own visual style . . . let it be unique for yourself and yet identifiable for others."
—Orson Welles

Once I was armed with my new style information (not to mention all my new makeup and dress routines), I wanted to share my discoveries with everyone. I had that new-convert syndrome for sure. My years of feeling makeup and style inadequacies spurred on a new sense of "I have found the key and let me show you, too."

I quickly enrolled in makeup classes. Soon I was training others with my newfound skills. I began sharing my makeup information with my clients. After all, I knew intimately how any woman could feel a bit like a fish out of water when someone hands her a makeup palette and a brush, expecting a positive outcome. I wish I could report that, through my makeup blunders, I could speed up the learning cycle for my clients, but quickly I discovered that everyone's journey has its own timeline. My experience alone could not speed up their process. What I could do, though, was make the transformation more comfortable. I could break it down into small steps, the first step being color.

THE COLOR PALETTE

Color came into play right away in my new makeup business—in particular, the right color. How could my color experience fail to influence the way I taught makeup? I saw so many problems with the makeup color choices, in addition to application issues, for my clients. For example, so many blue-eyed clients came in to see me with beautiful blue eye shadow paletts. My goal as a makeup artist was to have the world see the gorgeous eye color of each of my clients, not eye shadow.

I had to turn to science for the cosmetic answers I wanted. In the science of color we look to the color wheel for our answers. The opposite colors on the color wheel actually pop the opposing color. Those opposite colors are called complementary colors. Opposites attract. So if I want to attract your attention to my client's eyes, then I need to surround the eye with the color opposite the eye color appearing on the color wheel. Blue eyes choosing blue shadow is not going to make my clients' eyes pop.

We must also look at the hue, value, and saturation of the colors we see in the skin, hair, and eyes:

- **Hue:** The name of the color, e.g., red, yellow, or blue.
- **Saturation:** The brightness or dullness of the color.
- **Value:** How light or dark the color is.

So how do I translate these colors I see into the makeup my client should use? It sounds daunting, but once I knew what colors I was working with, I understood color. How does knowing more about colors help me to understand color for makeup application?

The magic is that, once you know your colors, you can train your eye to see what works and what does not work for you. What colors add ten years to your face versus what colors give you a youthful glow? Knowledge of my true colors and my new way of seeing color have saved me from selecting the wrong clothes and makeup. It is easy to get dressed in the morning, and I love the savings to my bank account, since I actually wear what's in my makeup bag and closet. And this will happen for you, too!

In my beauty business, the color wheel became my personal assistant. I began to share my personal color assistant with all of my clients. The color wheel and applicable science always have the right answer. Once I showed my clients how it works, they relax into the comfort of choosing eye shadow shades that appear opposite on the color wheel from their eye color. So does that mean that the bright, blue-eyed client needs to choose orange on the color wheel? Well, yes, they could, but they can also choose a color with an orange undertone. Say copper or a henna brown. Beautiful!

NOT ALL COLOR SYSTEMS ARE CREATED EQUAL

I did notice a fair amount of clients who would arrive with their color fans that were produced years before when they had had their colors professionally done. You would think that they would be easy clients since they knew their colors, right? Wrong. What I found was that they were locked into that color fan and believed that the exact colors from the fan must be on their eyes and lips, not just in their clothes. They looked all right, but not great with that choice. My question was, why? I began to notice that the intensity of each client's eyes would dictate the intensity of the color choice that I wanted to apply. Many of the color fans that my clients walked in with had the wrong intensity of color suited to their eye intensity.

Now what do I do? I believe in the color system. Why, then, were some of my clients falling through the cracks when it came to the correct makeup color choices? My answer for choosing makeup was that there are not four seasons of color as we were taught, but twelve. What I mean by that is, if someone came to me and said they were a winter, and I looked at them and saw a very light eye and a soft intensity facial color intensity, the winter pallet was too harsh. If I took the hue (color) from the fan and reduced the intensity, then they looked radiant. My process worked for every client if I let the light, medium, or dark of their eye intensity or saturation pave the cosmetic way.

Suddenly a new need (and so an opportunity) presented itself to me. To really serve my clients well, I needed to have some formal training in color assessment. I searched for a program that would take all the aspects of color theory that I felt were crucial to produce a beautiful outcome every time. I wanted a program that took each client's eye color, skin color, and intensity into consideration when colors were chosen. I really did not want a seasons approach where, for instance, all "winters" wear the same color choices.

Many of the color assessment programs group their clients into very large, general color categories, and so every one shoved into those huge, oversimplified categories are given the same generic color fans. Yikes! So many people I saw were definitely living in the wrong season. To top it off, I felt that face- and body-shape proportions would need to be taken into consideration when choosing to put together a successful overall look. While other programs tell you that you are just like everyone else, I feel you are unique. We are *all* unique! We can't just indulge in the latest trends and hope for the best.

I'VE FOUND IT!

Quite accidently I stumbled on a company called DRES and its unique concept, the DRES System. I was thrilled! Finally I had found a process that looked at clients' skin, hair, and eye colors. Not just a one-dimensional color, but all of the colors found in each client's hair, skin, and eyes. I knew this was the program that I had been looking for.

The DRES System's forty-two Ultimate Colors Palette is the perfect vehicle for my clients to discover their unique coloring and simply guide them to the color shades and styles that would work best for them. The forty-two Ultimate Colors Palette makes it easy for each of my clients to style themselves like a pro. Each person has their perfect color palette. It appears naturally in skin sans makeup, of course. Look at your face without makeup. Your color map is right there.

GETTING UNDER YOUR SKIN

To find your way through the makeup maze, determine if there is a warm or cool undertone in your skin. I always recommend having this assessed by a professional, but if you are a DIY gal, I can offer a few tips to help determine anyone's color map.

Clean your skin and add moisturizer, but no makeup. Grab a mirror and seat yourself in natural sunlight. Make sure to use a room without any strong color on the walls. Choose a neutral-color painted room, otherwise an unwanted tone reflection may be reflected onto your skin. Purchase some felt squares of varied colors from a craft store or simply grab some various colored T-shirts and other garments. One at a time, wrap each item around your neck.

What are you seeing? Do you notice fine lines and wrinkles? Do you see dark circles under your eyes? What do the whites of your eyes and teeth look like? Finding the colors that actually work for you will diminish lines, wrinkles, and make skin look brighter. It's just the opposite effect for the colors you drape yourself in that don't work for you. It will become clear which colors allow you to shine.

To find your skin tone (not skin color, but the tone that radiates from anyone's skin), find the answer to the question: "Am I a warm or a cool skin tone?" That seems to be trickier for the DIY gal to see. One way is to drape yourself in the brightest white available, and then look at your skin. Does your skin seem to have a yellow cast, or does it have a pinker (blue) cast to it? This answer will help determine if you have a warm or a cool skin tone.

YOUR MAKEUP PALETTE

Once you know if your skin tone is warm or cool, choose your makeup color palette. If you find yellow in your skin, it has a warm tone. And if blue is found, your skin is cool-toned. With a blue undertone, your skin will look better in cool, sheer, bright colors. Those with a yellow undertone can lean toward warm, earthy shades. Study the makeup palette for the undertone found in your skin. Remember, colors like yellow can be cool or warm, so use your new way of looking at color to really see the undertone. If you still can't determine or see the undertones, by all means, hire a color stylist—preferably one trained in the DRES System, of course! A professional can help you stay in your color tone for choosing foundation along with choosing the opposite (on the color wheel) eye shadow color from your eye color. Staying within your unique color tones will paint a beautiful picture of you!

"Makeup is a powerful way to effectively reveal something unique about your inner self." —James Kaliardos, internationally renowned makeup artist

You may be asking, now that you have a grasp on your true colors, "What do I need in my makeup bag? How do I translate my colors to select makeup and pick a perfect makeup palette? The answer will vary a little, depending on your age and career: Are you a professional women or an outdoorsy, natural girl?

I do find that many of the items that we will be discussing are universal. First things first: nothing takes the place of good, healthy skin care. It is crucial to take care of the foundation of your beauty, and that is your skin. Healthy eating and plenty of rest, in addition to using a good moisturizer and sunscreen, are a must before any makeup application. Washing your face each and every night also needs to fit into your beauty routine. Strange, I know, to start a makeup chapter with taking makeup off—but it is vitally important to remove your makeup every day. Women (and men) can spot old caking makeup from a mile away and it's not pretty. Makeup is not a suitable cover-up for bad skin-care habits.

You may have a deluxe makeup bag filled to the top with all the latest have-to-have cosmetics. Or maybe you have a disorganized makeup drawer, complete with free lipstick samples from 1990 rolling around in six unflattering shades. Neither extreme works well. Scaling up or down with some key makeup items and tools that really work for you can be liberating. Here are some of my top makeup items to include in your bag and how to apply them.

MAKEUP MUST-HAVES

Concealer

For a bright and eye-opening look, nothing beats concealer. Remember that a little goes a long way; cover-up products work best if they are applied sparingly. For an under-eye cover-up, find a shade that best matches your skin tone. Choosing a shade that is slightly lighter than the color matching your skin works well to minimize dark circles under the eyes. What if what you are trying to conceal is not under your eyes? What works to conceal a breakout, for example? Since learning how to use opposites on the color wheel to bring out and pop a color, the good news is that opposing colors can neutralize, too. Bring on the color correctors!

Color-correcting concealers come in a variety of shades including yellow, green and blue, orange and purple. How do we use this fascinating cast of colors? For instance, a new bruise is quite purple. The opposite of purple on the color wheel is yellow, right? Using yellow concealer will cover or cancel the purple in the bruise. On the other hand, if the bruise is old, it may be yellow in color, so cover it with purple. Green is the opposite of red on the color wheel. So for a breakout that is a red spot, use green concealer. Are you falling in love with the science of the color wheel yet?

Here are some basic rules that apply to the actual concealer application for under the eyes. Start by applying a small amount of concealer just under the tear duct area. Using a synthetic brush (fingers don't work well for this product application), sweep the product down and out to the outside corner of the eye. Wipe off your brush if you feel there is too much product under the eye. Blend the concealer with a clean brush until the desired coverage is achieved. Lightly dust the area with finishing powder, which will set the cover-up—creams can travel as skin warms. At this point, continue to apply eye makeup. When you're finished with your entire makeup application, revisit that under-eye area, blending one last quick sweep under the eye just to make sure there is no creasing.

Foundation, Powder, or Tinted Moisturizer?

A smooth, clear, youthful complexion is a universal desire. So it makes sense that the most important makeup choice to make is about foundation. If you choose a foundation that does not match your skin tone, everything else you put on your face will be less than flattering. How to choose the ideal foundation? Coverage is the first question to consider. Application is second.

For example, foundations can be applied only where needed versus all over the face for lighter coverage. Let's explore some foundation and coverage options.

Tinted Moisturizer

A tinted moisturizer combines the benefits of daytime moisturizer along with some pigment coverage. The moisture tints offer a sheer, light coverage. A traditional liquid foundation typically has more pigment than a tinted moisturizer. Liquid foundations and tinted moisturizers can work on all skin types. One difference between tinted moisturizer and liquid foundation is that most liquid foundation formulas offer a variety of finishes. Light- or full-coverage products are offered by the major brands, in addition to matte, shine-free, or enriched formulas. The application of liquid foundations and cream products is very important. Remember "Connie Cosmetic"? So be sure to blend, blend, blend.

Powder Foundation

What if you want a foundation that is a powder? Mineral powders do offer the coverage of a traditional liquid foundation in a powder form. As a bonus, many of the mineral powders on the market contain a blend of oxides that offer a naturally occurring sunscreen. By nature, the titanium dioxide and zinc oxide help to protect the skin from the damaging rays of the sun by offering an SPF of 15 or more, depending on formulation. Mineral formulas are popular for their breathable properties and lightweight feel. To catch the mineral wave, many major brands have added loose mineral powders to their offerings and tout that they carry mineral products. Make sure to read labels when choosing a mineral powder foundation, however, as many of the lines have fillers like talc.

Your Formula Match

Choosing a formula is number one and should be followed by choosing a color. The perfect foundation must match your skin color—not lighter or darker than your natural shade. Choosing a poor color match can age you. For a little more color in your skin, always use a bronzer, and not with your foundation. Keeping your foundation color true to you will always be more youthful and flattering.

Blush

Looking at almost any child, the glow from their cheeks broadcasts health and beauty. That glow that a child radiates naturally is what we should strive for. What is the natural color that you produce in your skin when you flush? That is the blush color tone to choose. Do not choose bronzer as a blush. I know it is easy to grab one item and just swipe it all over. In the bathroom mirror, the bronzer can even look like a wonderful, healthy glow. However, in the bright light of the day, the truth is just the opposite. Unless the bronzer color is your natural flushing color, bronzers applied as blush are aging and harsh.

Blush should enhance your overall look, not overwhelm it. Be careful not to overdo blush or choose the wrong color. You can look clownish if you are too heavy-handed, although I feel no one should leave out this step from their beauty routine. Blush is the *life* we put into our look. Blush can be used to form contours, too. Where you place your blush can be just as important as the color.

I love the ease of the DRES System: I can determine exactly what your face shape actually is. Why would this be important to know? Your face can look either become hollow looking or too full just by placing your blush in the wrong areas.

If you have a long face, for example, apply your blush to the apples of the cheeks and extend the color outward toward your ears. That will help create an illusion of width in your face. If your face is round, apply blush just above the apples of your cheeks and blend it out toward the ear and up to create a narrowing of the face. Once you discover your unique face shape, your blush will be a contouring or minimizing workhorse.

Mascara

The eyes have it, and we want the world to know it. I have seen mascara listed as one of the top two items women would take with them if they were stranded on a desert island (following lipstick as number one). We have sort of a love-hate relationship with mascara. We hate clumps, raccoon eyes, and dried-out tubes. We love looking awake, sexy, and flirty with the perfect lash.

Curling lashes before applying mascara will go far in our desire to look wide awake. When choosing mascara, consider its formula. What are the results you are looking for? Do you want lengthening, thickening, or a waterproof formula? As far as application goes, always apply mascara to the top of the lashes first, before coming up and out with the mascara wand. Wiggle the mascara wand back and forth at the base of lashes for a thickening effect. Two coats are perfect—more will only clump.

"Lipstick is the fire that lights the face." I heard years ago when I started my makeup business, and it has resonated with me ever since. Sadly, I have no idea who said it. So lipstick or gloss is a must! Once lipstick is applied, we know the statement is true.

The challenge is finding the perfect shade. A good rule of thumb when choosing a lip color is to go no more than two shades darker of the inner lower lip color. Again, we see that intensity of color matters. Staying in your warm or cool color tone will create a look that will be in harmony overall.

How do you apply lipstick? First things first: make sure that your lips are properly cared for—chapped lips are unattractive. Apply moisturizer to your lips just as you do for your skin. Lips are delicate and must be treated with the same care as skin. Don't forget that there should be a sunscreen in your lip products or it should be applied before lip color. Lips also need exfoliation from time to time to keep them soft and smooth.

Once you're ready to apply lipstick, decide what you want to accomplish. Are your lips on the small side or do you feel that they are too full? Do your lipstick colors bleed onto your skin? The answers to these questions will dictate your application steps.

For example, if your lips are smaller, to make your lips appear fuller, line the outside of your natural lip line. Then, apply a deeper shade of lip color at the outside corners of the lips. Next, apply a lighter version of a similar shade of the lip color to the center of the lips.

To reduce the fullness of your lips, line the inner side of your lip line and then use a darker, matte shade of lip color. If your issue is lipstick bleeding into creases around your lips, be sure to line your lips with a neutral lip pencil that is close to your natural lip color. There is nothing worse than seeing a woman wearing a dark lip liner under her light-colored lip color. This is also an aging, dated look.

HOW TO BALANCE EYE MAKEUP

First, determine the map of your face. Look in a mirror. An easy face test to start with is eye spacing. When I look at a client's face, I ask myself, "Can I fit a third eye between her right and left eyes?" If the answer is yes, then I should consider that my client has wide-set eyes. If the answer is no, then I know that my client's eyes are close set. My choice for makeup is going to be different for these clients and every client—I want to bring balance to the face. Let's look at the five basic eye shapes and the best makeup application to enhance each eye shape.

Almond

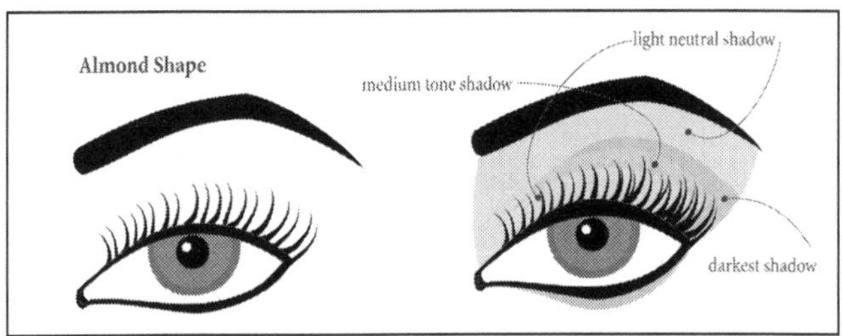

The almond eye shape is upswept at the outer corner. Use the following steps to help almond eyes appear larger and rounded:

1. From lash line to brow line, cover the entire lid with a light, neutral eye shadow.
2. At the crease line, apply medium-toned eye shadow; blend up toward the brow bone. Be sure to keep the color above the center of the eye.
3. Apply darker eye shadow to the outer third or corner of the eyelid, making a < shape with the eye shadow color. Then blend inward and upward.

4. Eyeliner on the upper lid can make almond eyes appear larger. For more rounded almond eyes, make the liner slightly thicker at the middle of the eye and then stop before the outer corner of the eye.
5. Shadow smudged on the lower lash line in the center of the lower lid will further round out the look.

Close-Set Eyes

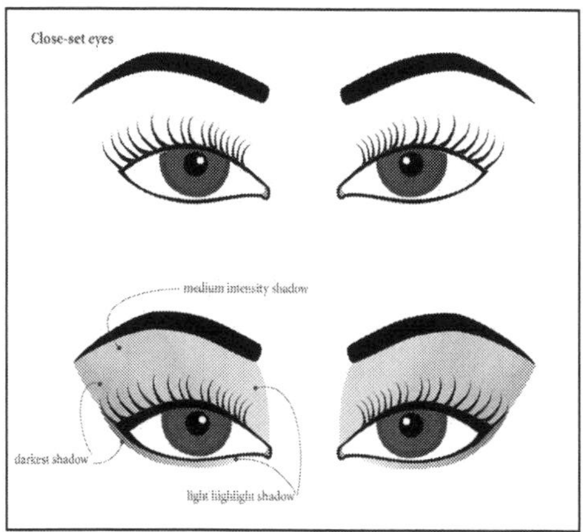

If the space between your eyes is shorter than the width of one eye, you have close-set eyes. With this eye shape, we want to create space between the eyes with the illusion of width.

1. Apply a light highlight color from the inside corner of the eye up to the brow bone.
2. Apply a medium-intensity eye shadow to the eyes' outer corners, from lash line up to the brow bone, and blend well.
3. Add a rich, dark color of eye shadow to the lash line, sweeping to the outer corner.
4. Line the eye. The liner should begin over the iris area of the eye and sweep out, extending beyond the end of the eye to maximize the lengthening effect. Keep the color concentrated toward the outside corners of the eye.

5. Smudge the darkest eye shadow shade onto the lower lash line from the iris line and out, keeping the inside area of the eye clear of the dark shadow.
6. Apply a highlighting shadow color to the lower lash area from the tear ducts area; sweep out to meet the dark shadow. (This area was kept clear of color in step 5.)
7. Mascara should be concentrated on the eyes' outer areas. For a special effect, artificial lashes can be applied to the outside corners. That will make the eyes appear even further apart.
8. Eyebrows should be tweezed slightly further out from the nose area to add space and create a more balanced look.

Wide-Set Eyes

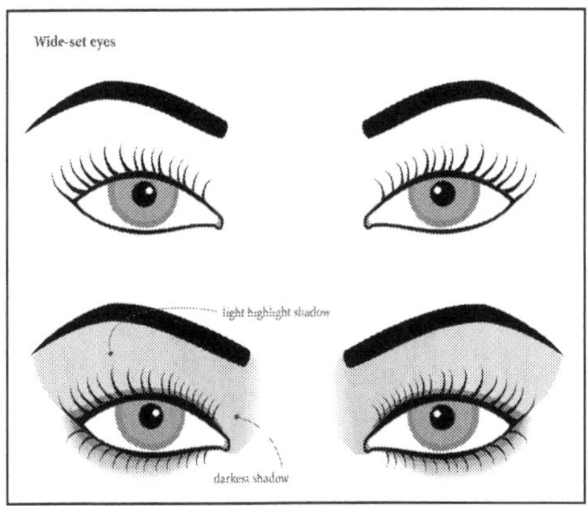

If the space between your eyes is greater than the width of one eye, you have wide-set eyes. The goal is make the eyes appear closer by eliminating some space, just the opposite of the close-set eye.

1. To minimize or reduce the space between the eyes, apply a dark eye shadow to the inner corner of the eyelids. Start the dark color in the tear duct area and extend it upward toward the brow bone and outward to the first one-third of the lids.
2. Next, apply lighter eye shadow to the outer two-thirds of the lid; blend upward to the brow bone.

3. Apply eyeliner to the entire eye. For a softer liner effect, use a dark eye shadow.
4. Mascara should be applied to the inner corners of the eyes, and out. If you want to apply artificial lashes, use a full strip or apply individual lashes to the entire eye.
5. Brows should be filled in closer to the nose to eliminate space and visually pull the eyes closer.

Hooded Eyes

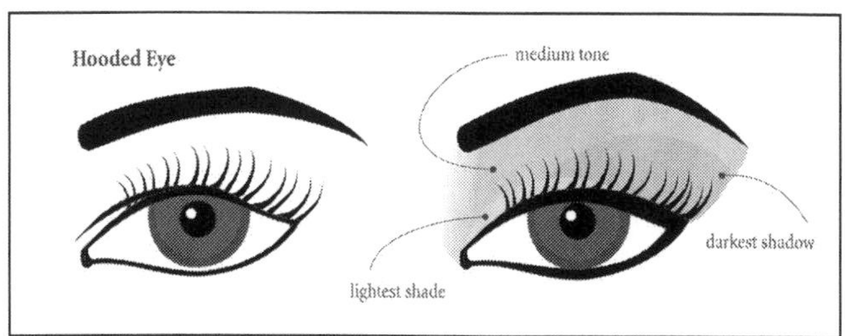

I like to call this "bedroom eyes." Think Drew Barrymore or Julie Christie. Many of my clients who have this eye shape are frustrated because they feel that their eyes appear to be partially closed. With this eye shape, the upper lid nearly covers the lash line. Many women feel that they cannot wear shadow on this eye shape. We can—by creating a crease.

1. Use a light highlight shade from the lash line to the brow bone.
2. Apply a shade slightly darker than the highlight shade over the outer third of the lid, and extend up to the area where you want to create a crease or indentation on the eyelid. Find this area by pressing gently at the top of the eye socket area and feeling where it naturally indents.
3. Use a darker contour shade on the outer corner, sweeping up and inward. Use a windshield-wiper motion to blend that darker shade in to create a crease.
4. It is important to use a liner to define the lash line of this eye shape.

The Prominent Eye

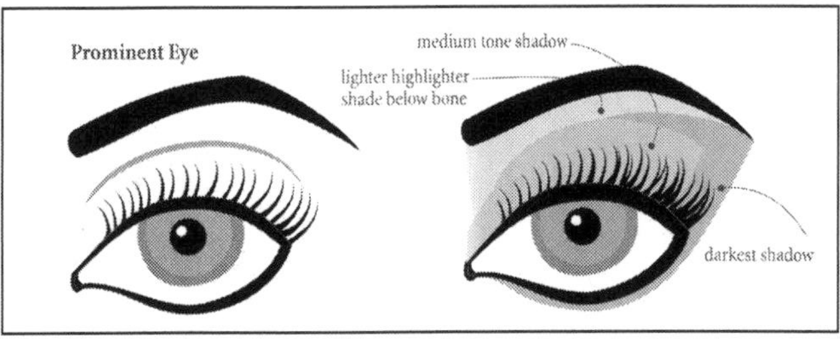

For this shape, we want to help reduce the prominent appearance of the eye and help make the eye appear as if it is receding rather than protruding.

1. Use a medium eye shadow shade and apply to the entire eyelid from lash line to brow bone.
2. Start at the lash line with a slightly darker eye shadow shade, and blend up toward the brow bone. Concentrate the darkest color near the lash line.
3. Apply the darkest color in the outer corner of the eye in a < pattern, blending toward your nose.
4. Stroke a lighter, highlighting shade under the brow bone and blend well.
5. Line the lash line with a soft, wider smudge of color, instead of a hard line, to add depth.
6. Line underneath your lower lashes.

SELECTING THE PERFECT EYE SHADOWS

If your eye color is:

Blue: Choose colors in the brown/orange family like warm, rich hennas or copper browns. Soft peaches or medium-to-bright orange and melon colors also work depending on your personal eye-color intensity.

Brown: Choose colors in the blue, green, purple, or charcoal ranges. Brown eyes can wear the largest spectrum of eye shadow colors. If there is an underlining accent color in your brown eyes such as amber, treat it as your color and accent eyes with the opposites of that shade.

Green: Choose pink and dusty rose shades if your green eyes are cool, and peach tones if the green tones are warm. Deep purples and soft violets will also pop and flatter green and hazel eyes.

EYELINERS

Depending on individual eye shape, eyeliners can lift the eye. Pay close attention to your eye shape when choosing how to apply eyeliner. Liner can change your look just by using different liner products. Liquid liner products give a more dramatic, defined look. A pencil liner can deliver a softer look. Whatever product you choose, be sure to apply the product deep into the lash at the roots. This will make lashes look thicker and will not show that strange distracting light gap between lashes and liner. Eyeliner underneath the eyes can often look harsh. If you like the under eye to be highlighted, try lining there with powder rather than pencil or liquid liner.

BEAUTIFUL BROWS

Brows are so important to a woman's overall look. They communicate so much and really accentuate any look. Brows can also offer an immediate eye lift. You can look younger and polished when your brows are groomed and cared for; think of the brows as a frame for the eyes. We would not hang a beautiful painting on the wall without an equally beautiful frame, would we? Don't leave your brows out of your makeup routine. They add expression to your face. Without brows, the balance of the face is thrown off, and beauty *is* balance.

I am asked daily:

- Where should my brows begin?
- How much of an arch do I need?
- Where should my brows end?

Here is a simple exercise to help you find the answers. Grab an eyeliner pencil and a regular long pencil or a straw. Line the pencil or straw straight up, starting at your tear duct area, extending it into your brow area. Put a dot where it lines up with your brow line. Does your actual brow start there?

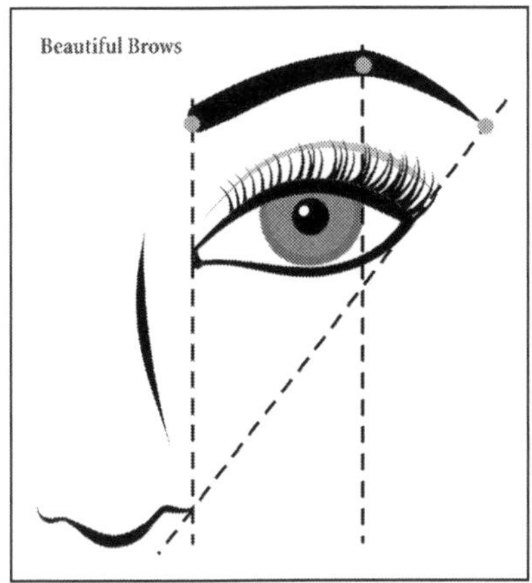

Next, the high point of your arch should be above the outer edge of your iris. Add a dot there. Take the pencil or straw and lay it from the outer nostril diagonally to the corner of your eye and into your brow area. Put your final dot there.

Step back and look at your result. Do the dots line up to where your brows are? Close? If your brow hairs extend beyond the dots, remove a few to attain a more natural and flattering shape. On the other hand, if brows are sparse, fill in the missing hairs with eyebrow pencil or powder.

There are several tools on the market to help achieve and maintain the perfect brow shape. Stencils are a great way to try on different brow looks. Choose a stencil that is in proportion to the structure of your face. Most stencil sets have a few different shapes to try. Choose the one that most opens up your face.

Use these "how to" examples to perfect your beauty statement. Give yourself some time to practice.

IS WHAT YOU SEE WHAT YOU GET?

Our looks affect us daily. Along with women, men are realizing this fact, too. That could explain why men are now having many of the cosmetic surgery procedures that at one time were used largely by women.

You are selling yourself daily at work or while looking for work, so your outward appearance needs to effectively represent what you have to offer. When I consider the reality of this perception, I see why anti-aging ads and products garner our attention. Gravity is always on duty and hard at work on our faces and bodies 24/7. I look in the mirror these days and my mother's jaw and neck are reflecting right back at me. When did that happen?

I remember reading the non-fiction book *I Feel Bad About My Neck* by Nora Ephron. The book was hilarious, and I laughed my way through it.

Sadly, I'm not laughing now. In my younger years, I ignored my neck when I applied moisturizer and sunscreen. The result is a very old neck. Oh, well! There's no time machine parked in my driveway, so if it really bothers me, it's up to me to find an anti-aging treatment or technique that can make up for years of neglect.

BOP! BAM! KAPOW!

Aging can sucker punch even the most confident of women. We have a daily ever-changing palette to work on. A brown spot pops up where there was none or we notice a new crease. The changes can be overwhelming. How we adjust to this time of our lives can be empowering, really. Don't fall into the trap of comparing yourself to other women, feeling insecure if somehow you feel you don't measure up. Maybe you feel you look much older than friends your age. Or you check out all the magazines and compare yourself to the models on the pages.

This sort of thinking leads us to make some very bad choices. While plastic surgery is fine, it can become an endless quest without boundaries. I have seen the most gracious and beautiful women alter their appearances and end up going too far. Some are never satisfied with the way they look and continue with one fix after another. Enhancing ourselves with makeup or cosmetic surgery can help us be perceived in a better light. But too much makeup or surgery—used to mask the real you—can be damaging to your overall image and others' perceptions of you. Makeup and cosmetic surgery should enhance and better express the real you to the world. Good makeup sharpens the focus and can allow you to naturally feel better about yourself.

Before you can express and highlight your best features, you must honestly know what those are. The truth is that our brains are more powerful than our eyes. What you see or think can vary wildly from day to day. After years in the beauty business, one thing I am sure of is that we do not really *see* ourselves. We look in the mirror every day; however, we fail to *see* our own natural beauty. Actually, many of us are uncomfortable with our natural beauty. I would bet that some of you are cringing right now, thinking, "I have *no* natural beauty." Are you stuck in that belief?

Time and again I see women who have handed over their beauty power to one facial feature that they see as flawed. They spend all their energy focusing on or attempting to mask that feature, ignoring their overall beauty. Compliments from friends or family do little to shift the focus from the perceived flaw to the beauty that is there.

This can be the type of thinking that takes a woman into the land of makeup overuse. Allowing your brain to get comfortable with your natural look is the first key to using your makeup appropriately—and aging well. The first and most important key to an anti-aging transformation with makeup is to look in the mirror with a bare face and love what has always been there.

FOUNTAIN OF YOUTH?

What are some anti-aging makeup marvels that we can explore and believe? The good news is that anti-aging makeup is from the beauty rule book that we already know. Our focus and techniques simply shift to a few different areas.

Eyebrows

Brows are the frame around the beautiful picture of our eyes. How your eyes are framed will add or subtract years. You may find that your eyebrows have thinned, possibly from youthful over-tweezing, and now your eyebrow hairs have stopped growing. The first reaction may be to tattoo or color in your brows where they used to be. Be careful. Choose a natural-looking, soft color to fill in your brows. Taupe is a good universal color for most women, in a light, medium, or dark taupe shades. If you do tattoo your brows and feel they look too harsh, lightly stroke the permanent brow with taupe pencil to create hairlike impressions that will soften the harshness. Comb the strokes with an eyebrow brush to soften them slightly to perfect the brow.

Teeth

Teeth give away our age—they dull over the years. According to the American Academy of Cosmetic Dentistry, teeth whitening is the most requested cosmetic dental service. Teeth whiteners are a definite anti-aging procedure.

Can you go too far with whitening? The answer is yes. The color in your eyes should dictate how white to lighten your teeth. It is really strange to see someone with those neon-white teeth: they look so unreal, and it's not a flattering look.

Fortunately, there are some options for lightening teeth. A dentist can safely apply a professional-strength whitening treatment, or at-home lightening strips can be used. The key is to stop when the white of your eyes balance with the white of your teeth.

Lips

Our lips naturally thin as we age. If you had a nice full lip all your life, you may not notice a big change. However, if you have always had smaller lips, this loss can be noticeable with aging. Some of the fixes can age us more. What is a woman to do? Lip augmentation with injectables, such as JUVÉDERM®, is a popular procedure and usually lasts about six to eight months. This can be the answer for some, but we have all seen this procedure overdone by some famous actresses. If this is a direction you'd rather avoid, what else is available?

Hydrate and moisturize lips. Hydration will add volume. When choosing a lip color, keep it on the natural, lighter side. Lighter colors make things look bigger. Those dark shades that we wore in our younger years can minimize the size of lips. The dark lip line outline is a huge makeup *don't* at any age.

To start your lip makeup application, brush foundation lightly over your lips. Line your lip with a nude-colored lip liner pencil on the outside lip line, close to your natural lip line. To enhance lip size, pay attention to defining the Cupid's bow of the upper lip with the pencil. White eyeliner or a white powder blended in above the Cupid's bow can give the illusion of a bigger upper lip. Make sure to blend it well. If you can't perfect this and end up looking like a "Got Milk?" commercial, skip this step. Finish off lipstick with a bit of gloss in the center of your bottom lip for even more effect.

Foundation

As we see those fine lines and wrinkles pop up, our tendency may be to cover them. Be careful! This is how we overdo our looks and age ourselves. We do want to soften our faces and, yes, cover our uneven skin, dark circles, and other imperfections. Can it be done without accentuating lines and wrinkles? Using very little foundation, not more, is the answer. Just cover the redness and imperfections. Otherwise, we may start to mimic Connie Cosmetic. Choosing the correct color shade for foundation is one of the biggest anti-aging tips I can offer. Again, wearing a too-dark shade, or a shade that is too pink or yellow for your skin color and tone, is the easiest way to age yourself. Choosing the correct makeup shade and formulations with light-reflecting properties will add to the moist, dewy look that says youth.

What about the "jowls" that we hate? The answer is to define the jawline. Apply a matte bronzing powder that's one to two shades darker than your skin tone under your jawline. From ear to chin underneath your jaw, blend this darker shade until you create a blended, shadow effect. (Contours should always be carefully blended so that they are not obvious.) This will create a nice sharp line, giving you a thinner, more sculpted face.

GRAY HAIR

Should we go gracefully through life with our graying hair or fight it? My answer is mixed and depends on how your gray hair makes you feel. Does gray hair make you feel washed out and tired? If your answer is yes, I would say color it.

Gray hair, however, can be gorgeous! Making the decision to go gray can be a relief for many women and can be very liberating. Jamie Lee Curtis has beautiful gray hair in addition to one of my favorite stars, Helen Mirren. What should you consider before taking the leap into a dramatic new shade? Tone—there is that word again! Everything comes down to tone, your tone. Cool gray hair shades have an ash tone whereas warm gray tones include yellow or gold. What tone will your gray hair cast? Will it suit your skin tone?

That is the issue we need to deal with as we gray. The wrong color tone in gray hair can make skin appear dull. Many times the early gray color has a pigment tone that changes over time. Until that happens, you can work with your stylist to highlight or change the tone of your gray hair. Keeping your gray hair vibrant and shiny is crucial as an anti-ager. There are shimmer-highlighting shampoos and leave-in sprays on the market to bring your gray hair to life. Gray is glamorous and sexy! Embrace it.

FINDING YOUR MAKEUP AND COLOR PERSONALITY

I encourage you to experiment and find your own makeup and color personality:

- Express *your* sense of self; it is not about conforming to someone else's style of beauty. Expressing yourself as well as flattering your figure is easy when you discover your unique code.
- Bring your features to life, and you will feel confident and, yes, powerful.
- Wear color with confidence. Smile often—nothing is more beautiful than a smile.
- Toss out some of the old beauty rules learned years ago and explore, experiment, and have fun with makeup.

- Check yourself and see what you are saying to the world with your makeup. Decide first what you want your first impression to be and apply makeup accordingly.
- Wearing the correct makeup will communicate to others that you give attention to detail and that you care about yourself.

LIPSTICK AND WORLD PEACE?

The thought I would like to leave you with is about the word *radiant. Webster's* definition refers to sending out rays: to shine brightly directly from the *center*. I urge you to find your center, your beauty balance. As I wrote earlier, beauty is balance. Feeling good about how you look increases confidence, which can lead to unbelievable life changes. When you feel better, you treat others better; happy, confident people contribute in a positive way.

Can I go so far as to say a little lipstick can change the world? I'd say the right shade of lipstick can change your world. So pucker up, and pass on the good feelings.

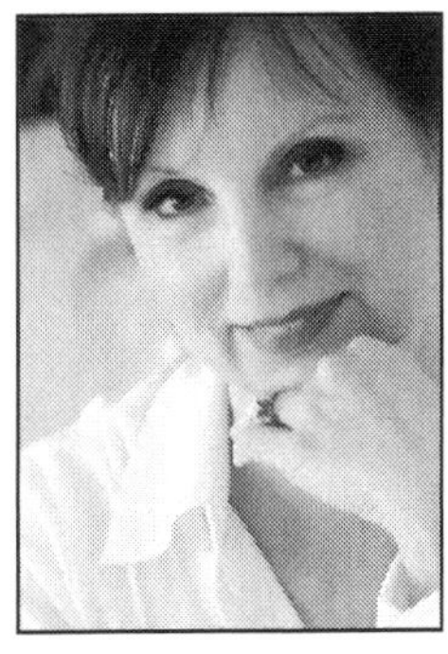

Brenda Azevedo

DRES System–Certified Personal Stylist

just B Cosmetics
www.justbcosmetics.com
brenda@justbcosmetics.com
Sacramento, California

Brenda is the founder and owner of just B Cosmetics, a custom blending makeup bar located in Sacramento, California.

With more than twenty years in the beauty business and as the former owner of an award-winning day spa, Brenda brings her significant hands-on experience directly to her work. Brenda shares this expertise with her clients to help positively impact how they feel about themselves.

Brenda's specialty is matching women with the perfect foundation shade and customizing formula for the individual's unique colors and skin type. Her beauty philosophy is "Be one in a million, not one of a million."

At the just B Cosmetics studio, Brenda helps her clients discover their best color combinations from the DRES System's forty-two Ultimate Colors Palette. Colors are chosen to complement skin, eyes, and the unique personality of each client and a custom DRES Colors Palette of forty-two Ultimate Colors is created, complete with a personal StyleGuide.

An individual DRES System face-shape assessment offered by just B Cosmetics uses a detailed formula to assist each client when they want to choose their best hairstyle, eyeglass frames, and accessories that will balance and accentuate their unique facial shape.

Brenda is passionate about teaching and sharing this makeup and color philosophy, and developing the tools women need to do this with ease! Brenda conducts beauty workshops around the country and mentors other makeup artists. She is also an author for *My Style, My Way*, a beauty consultant for BlogTalkRadio's "The Fitness IQ," and has received the "Best Makeup" Award from Sacramento's KCRA Television's A-List two years in a row.

CHAPTER 9

TIMELESS

THE ART OF AGELESS STYLE

By Cheryl Michaels

In the mid- to late 1960s, I was an awkward adolescent girl who dreamed of growing up and looking like an adult woman—and the sooner the better! I aspired to have the womanly beauty, elegance, and grace that I saw in my Midwest hometown of St. Louis, on television, and in fashion magazines.

When attending a special event, such as a theater performance or a wedding, where women were present, I always noticed them and how polished and together they seemed. They were glamorous in comparison to how I saw myself. I looked forward to the time when I could emulate their grown-up beauty and attractiveness.

I like to think I have had a reasonable amount of success at evolving through the years into a woman of confident style. Like many of us, I've definitely made my share of fashion blunders throughout the decades but all in all, it's been a satisfying and enjoyable journey.

I recently heard Joan Rivers on her snarky (albeit entertaining) cable TV show, *Fashion Police,* criticizing nineteen-year-old Miley Cyrus for looking "too old" on the red carpet at the Academy Awards. (Keep in mind that Joan also harpoons adult women of all ages for trying to look too young, so at least it goes both ways with her.) Joan sniped that Miley's hair, makeup, and dress were all too mature for her, and that young females should dress as young as they can, while they still can, "for heaven's sake!"

In my opinion, Joan's ageist assessment was unfair and off-base. Miley looked refined and sophisticated. I could relate to her desire to be styled as a woman, not a girl, for the internationally broadcast mega-event. A few months after the awards ceremony, Miley turned heads by wearing a double-breasted, white tuxedo jacket to the *Billboard* Music Awards. The problem was she didn't wear anything else besides a delicate gold chain and stilettos. Maybe she heard what Joan Rivers said about her Academy Awards "mature look," and she overcorrected. In all fairness, it's tough figuring things out when we are young. Being a celebrity in the spotlight certainly ups the pressure.

"There are only two ages: girlhood and womanhood."
—Christian Dior

When you were experiencing your transition from girlhood to womanhood, did you wish you looked older, sophisticated or even, dare I say, elegant? Did you admire actresses or other high-profile women of the time? Does anyone come to mind?

I immediately think of Catherine Deneuve, the face of Chanel Nº 5 in the late 1970s; Candice Bergen, former fashion model, actress, and comedienne on TV's *Murphy Brown*; and Jacqueline Kennedy, our beloved former FLOTUS (First Lady of the United States), who later became Jackie Kennedy Onassis and continues to inspire women all over the world.

I looked up to these women with awe because I could see their chicness and undeniable mystique—their actual ages had nothing to do with it. I honestly don't remember thinking about a glamorous woman's age when I admired her from afar.

Did you prefer reading grown-up fashion magazines such as *Vogue* or *Harper's Bazaar* over *Seventeen* and other teen magazines targeted for your age group? I think there are a lot of us who can relate to feeling a little cheated or left out back then, and I think there are also a lot of us who are still proud to stand up today and claim our womanhood.

As a DRES System Stylist, I don't advocate deliberately trying to look younger (although, hooray when that happens!) but, rather, knowing how to look youthful, stylish, and confident, regardless of your age.

This is not just a fantasy! Role models like Sandra Bullock, Helen Mirren, and Meryl Streep remind us that it's quite possible to look grown up *and* youthful. All three of these women are current Academy Award winners. Sixty-two-year-old Meryl Streep recently graced the cover of *Vogue*, making her the oldest *Vogue* cover model in that venerable fashion magazine's history. Newsstands are seeing a boom in baby boomers on magazine covers.

The Oscar nods to Sandra, Helen, and Meryl, along with the *Vogue* magazine cover, signal that a fantastic trend is under way. Our nation's fascination with youth is changing, and Hollywood is seeing a movement toward the authenticity of aging.

It's about time that such a shift would occur. It was destined to happen eventually. Fashion cycles come and go, as old becomes new again.

What causes consumers to become bored and want something different? The market becomes saturated by trends and fads, and we want something that feels new, even if it isn't. Apparently, we have become bored by our fascination with youth in our culture and a natural cycle is occurring.

It can't be denied that the baby boomers, those born roughly between 1946 and 1964, are a dominant U.S. demographic that is not only bored with what the media is feeding us but also impatient seeing only extreme youth everywhere we look. In the '60s, we were the hip and liberated generation of sex, drugs, and rock 'n' roll. We tended to think of ourselves as special, very different than those who had come before. As the empowered boomers move closer and closer to retirement age, we simply aren't willing to just fade into the wallpaper. I think we are collectively saying:

> *"I'm mad as hell, and I'm not going to take it anymore!"*
> —Howard Beale, in the 1976 feature film *Network*

I was riveted when NBC's morning show *TODAY* featured a segment in March 2012 about changing attitudes toward aging and beauty. A guest was the very attractive, seventy-two-year-old Valerie Ramsey. Valerie is a woman who was recruited by a San Francisco modeling agency at age sixty-three, and who has also been signed by an up-and-coming agency in Paris,

France, that represents male and female models aged forty through eighty-five.

The *TODAY* Show piece also spotlighted Iris Apfel, the flamboyant ninety-year-old New Yorker well known for her outrageous panache, who had become a new face of MAC Cosmetics. MAC said they chose Iris in response to customers looking for real representation. And for MAC to use a ninety-year-old model says that MAC is not afraid of the fact that a woman at *any* age can be really beautiful.

Clearly, MAC's gutsy choice, like their cosmetics, was right on trend—their highly anticipated Iris Apfel limited-edition makeup collection sold out within days.

The flamboyantly outspoken Iris told us: "Coco Chanel once said that what makes a woman look old is trying desperately to look young. Why should one be ashamed to be eighty-four? Why do you have to say that you're fifty-two? Nobody's going to believe you anyway, so why be such a fool? It's nice that you got to be so old. It's a blessing."

The modeling agency in Paris representing men and women ages forty to eighty-five, the aforementioned Hollywood movement toward the authenticity of aging, and the choice of Iris Apfel as a new, striking face of MAC cosmetics all indicate that a welcome shift is under way. This trend is encouraging, but more importantly, every woman can learn to assert her self-confidence, style, and individuality while looking current and relevant.

Relevance is a vital concept. It means that you are connected to the world around you and that you are dialed in to life. Many women, me included, have begun to feel more and more invisible. As we mature, it becomes more challenging to feel seen and heard. If you are a woman who was accustomed to receiving attention or being noticed, you may have slowly become aware that others seem to be looking right past you, as if you are irrelevant or invisible.

As the years went by, my frustration turned into apathy. Frustration caused me to give up and not care anymore, to become exhausted by the ongoing struggle to feel good about my appearance. It can be really exasperating for my generation of women to search for clothing that isn't too trendy and doesn't make them look like fashion roadkill, or even worse, *matronly!*

As a personal stylist, I have learned from my DRES System teacher Margaret Spencer that using the dreaded word *matronly* to describe an item of clothing will cause a woman to drop it like a hot potato.

IT AIN'T OVER YET!

DRES System Stylists have strategies and tips to bolster your confidence and help you get excited about being a woman again. I know this personally because the DRES System changed my outlook and attitude, and I have noticed a difference in how I am being perceived by others. The DRES System gave me fresh tools that have made clothes shopping fun again. I went through a phase when I didn't enjoy shopping and my wardrobe naturally suffered as a result.

It may sound a little superficial, but life is more enjoyable when we feel good about how we are showing up in the world. We all feel happier and more positive when we are having a good hair day. The same thing happens to our mood and 'tude when we know we are rockin' our style. I know this from personal experience. As I told a friend recently, "I no longer feel invisible," and that is an uplifting and empowering feeling.

As a DRES System Stylist, I want to give the boot to the concept of "age-appropriate" dressing and spread the idea that every woman can develop her individual style that is unique and vibrant without a date stamped on it. Women resent being lumped into age ranges, such as "over forty." This isn't fair, anyway, because it really doesn't tell us anything. Is that "over forty" woman forty-two or eighty-two?

Some of the most popular and famous well-dressed women over forty include Halle Berry, Sharon Stone, Annette Bening, Marisa Tomei, Oprah Winfrey, Jaclyn Smith, Michelle Pfeiffer, Glenn Close, Diane Keaton, Goldie Hawn, Jane Fonda, Diahann Carroll, Judi Dench, Celine Dion, Susan Sarandon, Ellen DeGeneres, Mary Steenburgen, Vanessa Redgrave, Lauren Hutton, Diane Sawyer, and Barbara Walters.

Most of us know that wearing clothing that is intended for a woman twenty to thirty years younger isn't the answer, and will only make you look older. We have all felt that odd discomfort when we perceive a woman's age anxiety, yet she hasn't said a word. What she is wearing betrays her.

So what *is* "ageless style"? It's finding the right clothing that suits your fashion style, and dressing consistently within that style. You do need to know the parameters of your style and what to look for. While you want to stay current, you shouldn't be scanning the racks looking for the hottest trends. Fashion is created to go out of fashion. A woman with ageless style is looking for the right pieces within her consistent style, her body shape, and in her ultimate colors.

"Fashion fades, only style remains the same."
—Coco Chanel

Discouragement has caused many mid-life women to give up or let themselves go. Letting go is a wonderful thing when it doesn't mean that you have stopped caring about your appearance, but it means that you have let go of the unrealistic expectations that our society and the media have heaped onto all women of all ages. Your DRES System Personal Stylist can help you overcome the apathy or, worse yet, negative feelings that so many women seem to have about their appearance.

FINDING YOUR STYLE

It's difficult to overstate the importance of confidence in all of life, but also when it comes to personal style, it's impossible to have it if you are playing it safe. Confidence is a key component in developing your sense of who you are and proudly showing it to the world. What makes you interesting is your unique idiosyncrasies, so don't be afraid to let people see who you are.

We are all growing and evolving throughout life. Clothing is a reflection of your self-image. Some of us are happy with what we see when we look in the mirror, while others might see a reflection that no longer suits who they are now. Not to worry. It's never too late to start again with a fresh approach to your self-image.

Most of us care what other people think, so how do you want to look to others, and what can you realistically pull off?

For your personal style to be effective and attractive to others, it must have an ease about it. You want to look natural and not like you are forcing or faking it. After all, who has the energy or time to keep that up, anyway?

THE DRES SYSTEM PROFILES

The DRES System defines five fashion styles. You may combine two styles to develop your own unique look. The key is consistency! The five styles are:

Classic: A Classic woman is tasteful, gracious, and timeless. She is sophisticated, polished, and refined. Nothing flashy or tacky would ever suit her. Michelle Obama, Cate Blanchett, Meryl Streep, Candice Bergen, Jennifer Garner, Diane Sawyer, and Katie Couric are Classics.

Chic: The Chic woman is modern and stylish. She is self-assured and dresses with confidence and flair. She likes to know what the trends are, and finds ways to integrate them into her wardrobe in a subtle manner. Jennifer Aniston, Anjelica Huston, Halle Berry, Angela Bassett, Sharon Stone, Julianna Margulies, Helen Mirren, Catherine Zeta-Jones, and Marcia Cross are Chic.

Romantic: The Romantic style is pretty, feminine, and soft. Romantics are friendly, casual, and whimsical. If you are a Romantic, you prefer girlish dresses over tailored slacks and lush sweaters over structured jackets.

Diane Lane, Ashley Judd, Kristen Chenoweth, Goldie Hawn, Meg Ryan, Andie MacDowell, Jane Seymour, Geena Davis, and Natalie Morales are lovely examples of Romantics.

Ethnic: The women who identify with the Ethnic style are authentic, diverse, and cultural. They are unique and interesting, and sometimes lean toward offbeat. They can also be hip, edgy, or bohemian. Famous women of this style are Iman, Barbara Streisand, Madonna, Diane Keaton, Whoopi Goldberg, Gwen Stefani, Meg Ryan (a combination of Romantic and Ethnic), Sheryl Crow (a combination of Chic and Ethnic) and Cher (a combination of Ethnic and Dramatic).

Dramatic: The Dramatic woman has a strong and exciting image. She is highly confident and knows what looks glamorous and striking on her. She loves to stand out, and is willing to invest the continual effort required to pull off this look day after day, year after year. Angelina Jolie, Celine Dion, Jennifer Lopez, Sophia Loren, Kim Basinger, Penelope Cruz, Tina Turner, Beverly Johnson, Ellen Barkin, and Oprah Winfrey (a combination of Classic and Dramatic) are examples of this dazzling female style.

THE KEYS TO THE KINGDOM OF BEAUTY: BALANCE AND CONFIDENCE

"Beauty is found in balance and confidence."
—Margaret Spencer, DRES System Creator and Founder

Women with ageless style have evolved over time and possess hard-earned wisdom, as well as both inner and outer beauty. They are disciplined in life and in their approach to their personal presentation. No matter how many gifts God has bestowed, it still takes effort to look your best, and women with ageless style have made that commitment. You won't hear them saying that they don't care how they look or that they have given up. Just because Ageless Style Women (ASW) make it look easy, don't be fooled into thinking they just roll out of bed looking pulled together.

ASW know who they are, and they own it with confidence and consistency. They take pride in themselves, and it shows. They project an intentional, authentic image. They are instinctively comfortable standing out as individuals by differentiating themselves, and might even be considered nonconformists. They are comfortable in their own skin. They know to avoid the "it" handbag and those big-lettered logo sunglasses that are so aging. If sunglasses have C's, D's or G's at the temple, just say no.

ASW wear their clothes; their clothes don't *wear them*. You'll never see a woman with ageless style in anything that looks silly or costumey. Overly bold patterns (geometrics or loud florals), wide stripes or childish polka dots just won't cut it. They also know that small prints can look too precious and are best on an apron or tablecloth. ASW run from anything that might be "sooo cute!" And that includes puffy sleeves or baby doll *anything*.

ASW strike a balance between being underdressed and overdressed and believe that, if push comes to shove, it's better to be slightly overdressed than underdressed (which is so not cool!) for social gatherings. Being a little overdressed is actually a compliment to your host. It says you respect the occasion and care enough to really show up for something you anticipate will be special. Being underdressed says you are either clueless or that "frankly, my dear, I don't give a damn."

ASW KNOW HOW TO BALANCE ELEGANCE AND SEXINESS

A classic rule to remember is not to wear tight with tight or baggy with baggy. If you are wearing a more body-conscious top, then choose a looser bottom piece. If your top is loose or blousy, then always opt for a more fitted bottom. Let one piece balance out the other.

ASW show skin strategically, knowing that men are visual creatures and have no problem visualizing what they can't actually see. In fact, I'm pretty sure most men wish more women would give them credit for that and leave a little more for them to imagine. Easy does it when it comes to showing too much skin, and a subtle hint of cleavage (if any), suits an ASW just fine.

A good rule of thumb is to show off only one body part at a time. Legs and cleavage is too much all at once—choose one or the other. ASW's clothing doesn't look as if they've been wrapped like a mummy but, rather, it gently skims curves. Their pants fall gracefully away from their bottom, and no cupping of cheeks is allowed. They reserve jeans with adornment on the back pockets for their daughters.

Diane Sawyer is elegant, intelligent, and desirable. Jaclyn Smith is gorgeous and refined, and men still find her irresistible. Susan Sarandon looks fresh and natural, and is an ageless, sexy favorite among gentlemen.

ASW also know how to dress down. After all, there is a time to pull out all the stops and a time to be casual and relaxed. A "casual uniform" can be very handy for running errands, your dental appointment, or shopping around town.

Save yourself time and energy by having several no-brainer, go-to outfits that you consider your knock-around uniform. Do you really want to have to think about this time and time again? Invent your wheel, and then run with it.

You can get scads of mileage from dark blue or black jeans, T-shirts, a couple of well-fitting jackets (leather or denim), and several scarves.

However, beware the denim leisure suit. Only one item of denim at a time, please. A denim jacket or vest with jeans is embarrassing to look at. When shopping for denim, remember that dark denim is more slimming than lighter washes. "Whiskers," which are permanent crease lines in the denim at the crotch level, draw the eye's attention to that area. Whiskers are for cats, not ASW.

When in doubt, go with the smaller size, as denim always stretches. For jeans that hold their shape, look for at least 2 percent spandex (such as Lycra). Look for heavier weight T-shirts, which are more forgiving of any little lump or bump than tissue weights. The magic formula for a soft and gently form-fitting tee is 95 percent cotton and 5 percent spandex.

Occasionally running around town in your fitness or yoga clothes isn't a fashion crime, especially if you are on your way to or from your class. Expecting a woman to go home in between her Zumba class and the post office just so she can change clothes is a bit much.

Just make sure you aren't paying homage to Jennifer Beals in *Flashdance*, or wearing an outdated nylon track suit, or those dreadful velour hoodie warm-ups that feature writing on your derriere. There are several popular lines of good-quality, flattering, stylish fitness clothes that are worth every penny, in my book: lululemon athletica and lucy activewear are my personal favorites.

DRESSING IN THE PRESENT

We want our image to fit the person we are today, not someone we used to be. We are interested in evolving as a person, while we simultaneously evolve our personal style. ASW know who they have become, and they stay true to themselves. They don't have time to wistfully hang out in the past when it comes to clothing or their body image. They aren't holding onto fuzzy memories. They realistically embrace the woman in the mirror, right now.

If you have arms that are toned enough for sleeveless, by all means, don't hesitate. If you have great legs that have withstood the test of time, show them off while you still can. (But anything shorter than an inch above your knee is too short.) Dress for your body as it is today, not the date on your birth certificate.

The two fundamental ageless style weapons a woman has in her arsenal are wearing quality clothing that fits properly and wearing the right colors for her skin tone.

If you don't have a tailor that you trust, ask your DRES System Personal Stylist or friends for recommendations. Expecting to be able to find clothes off the rack that fit you perfectly is pretty unrealistic. That expectation creates frustration, and will send you home empty-handed. A great tailor is indispensable to ASW, who know that using a good alterations person isn't too much trouble or too expensive. If you aren't knowledgeable about what magic your tailor might have up her sleeve, make sure an item is returnable in case she gives your newest item the thumbs down. It's also quite possible you have some great pieces in your closet that just don't fit properly. Your DRES System Stylist can help determine if a few nips and tucks will save the proverbial day.

Few women can afford to purchase an entire new wardrobe all at once. An effective strategy is to build on the good and better pieces that you have by adding current interpretations of the styles, shapes, and colors that are best for your personal style and body type. When you are shopping, always keep an open mind. Force yourself to bring at least one "I'd like this on someone else" item into the dressing room. Every now and then you are going to get a really pleasant surprise.

We all have color preferences, and we've all had time to figure out we purchased a color bomb at least once. You know, that blouse that always made you look like you were coming down with a case of botulism. As an experienced color consultant, I know that most people, men and women alike, are not very confident about their color sense. In fact, for many, choosing colors is about as much fun as an IRS audit.

So we understand that wearing the right colors is at the foundation of looking your best, yet only the lucky few who have been blessed with a natural eye for color know how to find their best colors without assistance.

When a professional color analysis is done by a certified DRES System Personal Stylist, she takes a close look at your skin in good daylight to determine your undertones. She is looking for the predominance of warm or cool tones. She will also observe your eye color and its varying shades and flecks, as well as the different shades in your hair. You may have had your colors analyzed in the past, but again, it's the present that counts. Just like your natural hair color has changed over time, so has your skin, whether it's been noticeable to you or not.

When your DRES Stylist finds the colors for your forty-two Ultimate Colors Palette, you will have made one giant leap toward creating the ageless style image that is so magnetic. I like to call them your *Wow* colors, because they are the colors that make me say "Wow!" when I hold them to your face during your color analysis. When you know your personal Wow colors, say good-bye for good to that color rut you might be in.

LET'S TALK ABOUT COLOR RUTS

Could you be a black-aholic? Black is the default neutral choice for too many women. I am currently in recovery from that affliction. Black absorbs light and will drain the color from your face and hair, making it a harsh choice for most women.

If you have a huge section of your closet that is dedicated to black, you are likely a "black-abuser." Fear not, though. We can do an intervention and leave that in the past.

That's not to say that black hasn't earned its rightful place as royalty among colors. It would be hard to garner support of a case to dethrone the little black dress as the one piece that every woman needs in her wardrobe. If you find yourself with too much black, though, and you can't afford to send it all to charity just yet, hold onto your cache of black a little longer with the clever use of scarves. Create a frame for your face with a scarf that has your ideal colors in it. This will instantly soften the negative effect that black has on your neck and face. It's a useful temporary strategy, but not a lifelong plan.

After black, white is the next most misunderstood and misused neutral. All whites are not created equal, and white is not the universal, no-fail color that we tend to think it is. Brighter, crisp whites look best against cool complexions. Creamier whites will make the warm-toned women come alive. Again, if there is a disproportionate section of white in your closet, use the scarf trick to get more flattering wear from your white clothing.

Monochromatic dressing, or wearing the same color from head to toe, is a timeless and chic approach. One color elongates the body because the eye moves seamlessly up and down. I especially like monochromatic outfits in neutral colors such as white, cream, camel, brown, navy, and olive. Pantsuits work particularly well in these colors.

AGELESS STYLE: BREAKING IT DOWN

The essential, classic items every ASW should own are:

Ballet Flats: An ageless classic with a chic and youthful flair. Ballet flats with a cap toe can be especially stylish. Best for daytime, of course, because the heels come out when the sun goes down.

Black Opaque Tights: Jackie O was a big fan and undoubtedly knew black opaque tights make legs look longer and sleeker, especially when paired with pointed-toe, black pumps. Spend the extra money it takes to get the best quality. You want the most opaque you can find because you don't want to see any splotches of skin through the tights. I was recently in an airport where I almost couldn't stop looking at a woman in her late fifties (I think!) who was wearing black leggings as pants. Unfortunately, they were *a little bit less* than entirely opaque. Occasionally, you might happen upon this fashion disaster: a woman wearing leggings as pants, which they most definitely are not.

Cashmere Sweater: Women have been remembering the cachet of cashmere since 1937 when Lana Turner wore a tight blue pullover version in *They Won't Forget*. Cashmere is the warmest of all natural fibers, and provides a feather-light feel without added bulk. Always elegant and timeless yet sexy, too! Cashmere is sexy because it is soft and feminine and will make the person you are with want to touch you.

Diamond Stud Earrings: I decided I like Barbara Walters when she admitted she wears cubic zirconium studs. That kind of honesty is refreshing and, if CZ is good enough for Barbara, it's good enough for me. It's almost impossible to do this earring, real or fake, the wrong way.

Maillot Swimsuit with Sarong: For years, I've been observing ASW poolside at upscale, glamorous resorts. I'm always a little dazzled as she glides to her sun lounger. There is a formula to this hypnotizing look: wide-brimmed straw hat, big sunglasses, black one-piece swimsuit, elegant sarong tied at her waist, metallic or beaded kitten-heel sandals, and a quality tote bag. Shake and pour.

Nude Pumps: Neutral and very versatile, every woman needs a pair of nude pumps in her shoe wardrobe. Look for a pair that match your skin tone as closely as possible and that have a pointed toe. They will elongate your legs and look much more stylish than black or white pumps.

Pearl Necklace: The pearl necklace was Jackie Kennedy's personal signature. She wore them when she married JFK, on the presidential campaign trail, and while strolling the avenues of Paris, Nantucket, and New York. Like diamond stud earrings, pearls can be real or they can be faux. Just don't use them too sedately, or your pearls will swing from classically cool to the thud of matronly faster than you can say Great Aunt Gertie.

Trench Coat: Can you visualize Meryl Streep in *Kramer vs. Kramer*? Even though Meryl has said that she "couldn't care less" about fashion, she is nonetheless a fashion goddess. She donned the classic khaki, belted trench coat with boots in her early days on the big screen in *Kramer vs. Kramer*. What a gracefully gorgeous, ageless woman she has always been!

Wellington Boot: Fashion meets function. Like Londoners, Seattleites are experts when it comes to practical options for a rainy day. Combine practical with classic style and you have the genuine winner, also known as Wellies. Hunter makes the original boot beloved by every Brit, including the royal family when they are just mucking about the palace grounds. Tuck slim, dark denim jeans into your Wellies, throw on your trench coat and mysterious sunglasses, and you will be well on your way to being followed by paparazzi.

FAVORITE AGELESS ITEMS

Belts: Belts were out of fashion for a while, but they are back in a very big way. Never underestimate the power of a belt to instantly transform a basic or even boring outfit. Jeans and a T-shirt come to life with the addition of a skinny, animal print number. Look for unusual designs, surprising colors or fabrics, and big, eye-catching buckles. Keep in mind, though, that belts need to be appropriate for body shape. This is something your DRES System Personal Stylist can help you with.

Denim Jacket: A casual fashion workhorse, this must-have piece just keeps going and going. The best version is dark and looks like it's been worn a zillion times. You want it to be fitted, not boxy or oversized. It shouldn't look like you are heading out to bale hay. Over a dress, it looks hip and current, especially if it's a bit body-conscious. Scour vintage shops for something retro none of your friends will have.

Driving Shoe: Two words: upscale leisure. More stylish than a basic loafer, the car shoe looks amazing with indigo or white jeans for classic elegance. Visualize Nantucket in the summertime, a red roadster convertible, and a scarf blowing in the wind. The next time I see a pair in suede or leopard print, I'm grabbing them.

Jeans: Best in dark denim sans embellishments or holes. ASW know to avoid adorned or very low-rise denim. Holes and rips look out of place on an adult woman. There is a reason why NYDJ—Not Your Daughters Jeans have been so successful. Always remember to check the rise, the distance between crotch and waistband, to make sure it isn't too snug or too droopy. And while you're at it, always check the rear view.

Leather Jacket: I have a simple, quilted Chanel-inspired leather jacket that I've had for years, and I get at least one compliment every time I wear it. The trick with a leather jacket is that you don't want to look like you are trying too hard. Epaulets, too many zippers, chains, or other over-the-top details will push you into the danger zone. Keeping it simple will keep it chic. Don't reserve your leather jacket just for casual wear—experiment wearing it over dresses and you just might pull off the almighty combination of powerful, edgy, and flirty.

Peacoat: Low-key, unpretentious, unfussy style; that's the time-tested peacoat in a nutshell. The fabric is a stiff wool and looks best in the classic colors of navy, black, gray, or forest green. A navy peacoat with slim jeans, your driving shoe, a scarf, and aviator sunglasses says, "I'm low maintenance, and I'm totally put together."

Plain White T: We've talked about not trying too hard because there is a certain unabashed ease to ageless style. Well, it doesn't get much easier than a three-pack of men's Hanes white T-shirts! What's not to love about a basic that you can pick up at Target? The Gap also carries quality, crewneck T-shirts for around $15.

Use the plain white T to dress down a pantsuit or add a fresh, modern flair to a conservative V-neck sweater. Make sure it isn't too tight or too short if you are wearing it alone with jeans or capris. T-shirts and pants have something in common: if you're wondering if they are too tight or too short, the answer is yes.

White Jeans: Dress them up or dress them down—white jeans look crisp and fresh in spring and summer. Basic straight leg or boot cut look best.

Avoid embellished or trendy versions. Try them with a chambray shirt, a soft blousy top, or a silky tunic.

Wrap Dress: Diane von Furstenberg created the holy grail of sexy, elegant dresses for women of all ages, shapes and sizes. The wrap dress is alluring without being sleazy and flatters every woman's figure because it hugs our curves and gracefully drapes at the same time. The original fabric was jersey, and this dress is a dream for traveling. Try it with knee-high boots and, of course, pumps and wedges.

I'M SEXY, AND I KNOW IT

Animal Print: Leopard, especially, is timeless, a little racy, and always throws a glamour punch. Just make sure your animal print is in neutral colors, not hot pink or lime green. If you aren't sure what good animal print looks like, as opposed to tacky animal print, check out the designer clothing, shoes, belts, or handbags at a high-end department store. Keep everything else simple and neutral.

Aviator Sunglasses: The aviator shape will never go out of style, period. It's classic and ageless, and they have a sexy *Top Gun* edge to them. Pair them with jeans, a plain white T, and a clean leather jacket, and you will nail the sweet spot of cool. Best to avoid the mirrored ones; it's oddly disconcerting to know that I could check my teeth for poppy seeds while I'm chatting with someone wearing aviators.

Boyfriend Cardigan: Menswear looks on women are undeniably sexy in a quietly well-dressed way, and the boyfriend cardigan is no exception. Try it belted over a T and jeans, or over a feminine dress. Red looks especially alluring.

Cape: Not just for Superman, a cape is the epitome of elegant sexiness, and will unleash your inner Wonder Woman. It's the perfect way to spice up tailored layers underneath and shouts, "I've got style on the fly!"

Chandelier Earrings: Captivating and decidedly feminine because of their movement and sparkle, chandelier earrings are a stand-alone statement, and generally should not be paired with a necklace. Opt for a bracelet or cuff instead.

Cowboy Boots: You needn't be from Dallas to know that a pair of cowboy boots worn *under* jeans (not tucked in) is a quick ticket to earthy female swagger. Spend the extra bucks for Tony Lama or Lucchese, and get your "Don't mess with Texas" attitude on big-time.

Fishnet Stockings: *Don't* be the woman who wears the seamed ones with high heels and a short skirt, but *do* be the woman who wears fishnets with a knee-length skirt and classic pump, or peeking out from the hem of tailored pants. You want the smallest net you can find, not the larger ones, and layering nude pantyhose underneath your fishnets is a slick trick.

Knee Boots: Powerful looking, tall boots hint at your inner bad girl and say, "I'm the one in charge here." They are at their ageless best when they hit just below the knee and your skirt or dress hits just above the knee. Try them with black opaque tights if you aren't crazy about showing your knees. Over-the-knee boots look trashy, and go-go boots will make you look like you are a channeling Nancy Sinatra. Best not to go there.

Mary Janes: It's the strap over the instep on a pump or slingback that creates the desirable Mary Jane. The most coveted version is the Manolo Blahnik Campari, with pointed toes. I wore out a pair of these a few years ago, and have decided I should start saving for pair number two. They were the most expensive shoes I have ever owned, and unquestionably my favorites. Most of the time, you really do get what you pay for.

Do you know what these are? Manolo Blahnik Mary Janes. I thought these were an urban shoe myth!
—Carrie Bradshaw in *Sex and the City*

Metallic Sandal: The metallic sandal rocks in flat thongs, gladiators, kitten heels, simple slides, or stilettos. Copper, bronze, silver, pewter, or gold. Matte, shiny, or textured. The metallic sandal is versatile and chic all summer long, and is especially great for parties and travel. I love them worn with a maxi dress.

Suit: When choosing a suit for work, look for one that will also work by breaking up the pieces. Can the jacket be worn with jeans, or the skirt with a leather or denim jacket? To make your suit more sexy for evening, add a lacy camisole (or no blouse at all if the first button is high enough) and a pair of stilettos, and your sexy sophistication will speak for itself.

WHAT NOT TO WEAR

Animal Print Overkill: Only one animal print item at a time, please, and no jungle-print spandex for the gym.

Baggy Bra: A good-fitting bra that lifts up the girls is the fastest way to instantly erase years and pounds. Nothing says *matronly* quicker than saggy breasts, and adding visible panty lines is a double whammy. There have been so many advancements in undergarments and shapers that there really is no excuse for doing yourself such injustice.

Bedazzled Bling: Sparkle, sequins, glitzy trim, or jeweled embellishments make others wonder if you've fallen prey to late-night infomercials. Beware the BeDazzled look.

Big Shoulder Pads: Linda Evans and Joan Collins wore BSPs for their famous catfights on *Dynasty*. That was in the 1980s.

Boring Coat: Never waste your money on a boring coat. Frequently during cold weather, your coat, shoes (or boots), and handbag are all that other people will see of you.

Boxy Jackets: You can do so much better than wearing oversized, boxy jackets intended to hide your figure. Your DRES System Stylist can show you how to make the most of your body type.

Clanging Jewelry: Too much jewelry; loud, clanging jewelry; or multiple rings say "crystal ball reader."

Costumey, Theatrical, Eccentric: These looks are best reserved for the very young. We all enjoy positive attention, but looking like Carmen Miranda just says "kooky and on my way to senile."

Dark Lipstick: This is a very common mistake. Dark lips are quite aging, and the antidote is a paler, softer color. Dark or neon nail polish and unnatural-looking French nails will draw attention to your hands and feet, two features that I choose to downplay. I diligently searched for a nude polish that closely matches my skin tone—it looks clean, modern, and ageless.

Fair Isle Crewnecks: Nor the dreaded holiday sweater. Ho-ho-ho is no-no-go. When a woman wears a holiday sweater to a party, she gives the impression she didn't have any idea what to wear—or maybe didn't care.

High-Water Pants: Wide-leg pants that are too short. These are sometimes spotted with Birkenstocks here in the Pacific Northwest. One of the biggest mistakes women make is wearing pants that aren't the right length for their shoes. Your pants should be hemmed for either flats or heels. Sorry, but you just can't have it both ways. Hems should just graze the tops of your shoes and be a half inch to three-quarter inches off the floor.

Limp, Lifeless Synthetics: The kinds of fabric for shirts or blouses that cause static electricity in your hair when you pull them over your head.

Metallic Emblems or Logos: Emblazoned on T-shirts or jacket pockets. That big lion head one comes easily to mind.

Orthopedic-Looking Comfort Shoes: If you really need to wear orthopedic shoes, that's one thing, but wearing those inexpensive, boring pumps we are all familiar with will add years to what otherwise might be an attractive outfit. Abandon your chunky and clunky mid-height or low heels after five o'clock. Just remember: After five, chunk goes clunk.

Prairie Prints: Girly pastel prints or any print that brings Laura Ingalls to mind will make you look like you are headed out to pasture.

Pleated Pants: Pleated pants are neither stylish nor flattering. And please be very careful about elastic-waist pants. Too forgiving, they can make you complacent and unaware that your waistline is expanding. Elastic waistbands are a slippery slope, and I speak from experience.

Queen Mum Handbag: Any handbag that looks like it should be on the arm of Prince Charles's mother should be donated to charity. Also, those multi-pocket organizer handbags are frumpy. Your handbag gives you another opportunity to say "I get it."

Rhinestone Readers: How do I know about rhinestone reading glasses? Because I own a pair that I impulsively bought back in the day. Now I leave them in my nightstand drawer for a late-night reading emergency. Steer clear of any eyewear, especially "granny glasses," that say glitz, whimsy, or "I'm fun." Your DRES System Stylist can analyze your facial shape and help you find a modern, flattering pair. You deserve it.

Ruffled, Lacy, Tiered Skirts: Or all of those together. Just walk away from handkerchief or uneven hems; we're back in "crystal ball reader" territory.

Tiny Jewelry: Small, dated-looking necklaces, like a little garnet on a thin gold chain, say that you are in an accessories time warp.

Ultrasuede: Ultrasuede harkens back to the 1980s when it was an exciting new invention. It reminds me of the first time I saw pleather and thought it was fascinating.

INAPPROPRIATELY YOUNG DANGER ZONE

Cheap-Looking Chains, Earrings, or Hair Accessories: Unless you are with your daughter or granddaughter, don't go in that accessory store at the mall for tween and teen girls. Also, anything from Forever 21, Bebe, The Limited or Express is off-limits.

Cotton Candy Pink or Neon Color: If the color has the brightness usually found only in cans of spray paint, it's better reserved for car wash or garage sale posters.

Leather Pants: Have you ever seen leather pants on a man or woman that didn't make them look like they were trying too hard to be hip? Fit is always problematic with leather pants, so their being too young is just the beginning of the reasons to rule them out entirely.

Motorcycle Jacket, Chains, Anything Shouting "Biker Babe": No explanation required, although I will acknowledge that there seems to be a preponderance of single, middle-aged men who ride Harley-Davidsons and would love to meet women who want to go for a ride.

Nosebleed Stilettos: Pass on any heel over three inches and those ankle-breaking platforms.

Rompers: I wore terry cloth rompers during hot, humid summers in the Midwest. I also wore tube tops. I was in my teens. It was long before answering machines, cell phones, and the Internet. We did have eight-track tapes and color television, though.

Shorts: Shorts are for children. Shorts do not flatter adult men or women and, in fact, Americans who travel abroad and wear shorts are considered to look foolish and tacky. The whole point of shorts is that they are supposed to be comfortable, but we have all seen many ill-fitting pairs of shorts on women whom we know couldn't possibly be comfortable. The pleated short is an especially egregious style *don't.* A skirt, capris, or a dress is a much better choice for an ASW than shorts. If you can't give up shorts entirely, opt for walking or city shorts.

Skinny Jeans: You know who you are if you can pull off this look. Regardless of age many women can't, but that shouldn't stop those who can. When skinny jeans first appeared several years ago, they were a bit shocking and seemed like a fad that wouldn't last. Now we are accustomed to seeing them, and the look still has legs. If you want to try them, a loose tunic top with gladiator sandals or wedges might work. Another option is a longer cardigan or coat-style sweater with your skinnies tucked into boots. This is an example of the previously mentioned "loose top piece with snug bottom" concept.

UGG Boots: Yep, they are cute and stylish, but middle-aged women were never the target market. UGG boots are sold in Brass Plum Shoes at Nordstrom. They shout "I share my daughter's clothes."

Victoria's Secret Pink or Juicy Couture: I'm always a little embarrassed when I see young women with the words "Pink" or "Juicy" stitched on their derrieres. To see that on an adult woman leaves me speechless.

AGELESS ACCESSORIES

Bold Items: Few things make a visual statement of personal style like costume jewelry. A prominent necklace, a big cuff, or an oversized, eye-catching ring all transform a simple look. Current-looking shoes (which doesn't have to mean nosebleed heels or mega platforms) that suggest a trend will add a welcome dose of ageless *now* to an outfit. Bold accessories instantly articulate a woman's sense of style.

Gloves: Gotta love 'em. Start with a pair of leather driving gloves. The ones with holes at the knuckles, or even the fingerless kind, will tell the world you have style *and* attitude.

Pashmina: Classic, feminine, and practical all at the same time. Great for travel, especially since commercial airlines don't provide blankets anymore.

Silk Scarf: I wasn't born knowing how to wear a scarf. In fact, I was "scarf-challenged" until I had a come-to-Jesus moment of inspiration when Margaret Spencer and I were experimenting with scarf tying. When you understand the beauty and versatility of scarves, you shall surely hear the angels singing.

Scarves don't have to be silk, and if you're not quite ready to adorn your neck with wild abandon, try tying a scarf onto your handbag. French women routinely do this, and it's *très* chic, *oui oui!*

Sunhat: A floppy sunhat with a ribbon band is always classic and ageless. A cowboy-style straw hat can also look very cool on a woman while she's riding in a convertible or lounging at the pool. I can't say the same about golf visors, which scream "retired." Save your golf visor for actual golfing.

Upgraded Buttons: Buttons can function like jewelry for your clothing. Sometimes an otherwise lovely garment will have very plain or cheap-looking buttons. Take a look in your closet and see if there might be a coat, suit, or jacket that could really come alive with beautiful buttons.

AGELESS STYLE = SELF-AWARENESS

Many women in their forties, fifties, and beyond have experienced changes, challenges, and losses. This can be a very tough time of life for women. There's menopause and other issues of aging to deal with. Weight gain, wrinkles, and gray hair can make us feel we have lost our attractiveness.

Add to that the empty-nest syndrome and the feeling of not being needed that we might struggle with. Some of us go through divorce or are widowed, while others have the need to look after elderly parents or have lost their parents.

Midlife and beyond is a time for women to feel comfortable about who they have become, to define and refine their own identity, and not the identity they have allowed themselves to embody based on others' expectations. The good news is that the maturity, strength, and wisdom they have gained, sometimes through loss, gives them freedom from youthful insecurities. That is one of the challenges of youth, wondering and worrying about how we look to others. Later in life, we are free to re-create ourselves in an image of our own liking. We are ready to please ourselves.

At the time I am writing this, baby boomers are roughly forty-eight to sixty-six years old and can anticipate living another thirty years or longer. The boomer generation is one accustomed to defining new ways of thinking. They did it in the 1960s and '70s, and they are going to do it again over the next few decades as they redefine aging.

Baby boomers are already changing how all of us think about the second half of life. They are physically and mentally more active, keep their professional lives longer, and engage in fulfilling personal pursuits more than we have ever seen in generations before. The boomers are going to defy biology as long as possible, and the movement toward the authenticity of aging will continue for at least the next fifteen, twenty, or even thirty years.

It's never too late to renew your commitment to yourself. If you are feeling overwhelmed, I don't blame you. I have been in that paralyzing place. When your DRES System Personal Stylist helps awaken you to your potential, your natural enthusiasm will take over and you will see *YOU* differently. And so will everyone else.

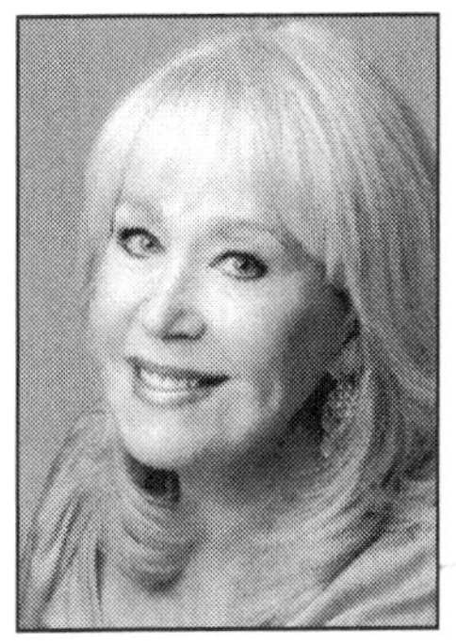

Cheryl Michaels

DRES System–Certified Personal Stylist

www.cherylmichaels.com
AgelessStyleCoach@gmail.com
Issaquah, Washington

Cheryl Michaels, CPC, is a certified professional coach and a DRES System–Certified Stylist. Coaching and styling allow her to express her passion for design and style while enabling her to help others. Her philosophy is that both disciplines rely heavily on good listening skills and asking thought-provoking questions, which lead to finding the answers and solutions that her clients are seeking.

Cheryl enjoys being a regular contributing writer for *Kalön Women* digital magazine, where she muses about a variety of topics of interest to women forty and over, *Kalön Women*'s target audience. She is particularly interested in the subjects of female life transitions and the reinvention of one's self. (The word *kalön* is Greek for beautiful.)

A favorite message of Cheryl's is that true ageless style starts with confidence. When that confidence has eroded for any reason, it reflects in a woman's external presentation, furthering the erosion of her self-confidence. So it is a circle of the internal reflected in the external and vice versa: a vicious cycle that is easy to fall into but can be broken with help from your DRES System–Certified Personal Stylist.

Over the years, she has been a small-business owner in the fields of landscape design and interior and exterior paint color consulting. Photography, hiking, and travel are her favorite pastimes, and she combines them whenever she gets the chance. Cheryl has two adult sons who both live in the Seattle area, where she also resides.

HOW TO GET DRES

Get your free DRES Profile at www.DRESsytem.com. Here you can join the DRES Club and get help online from our DRES System Certified Personal Stylists, or receive our newsletter to get free style tips. Our Personal Stylists can make recommendations on clothing to help you find a great fit in your private online showroom. We have DRES Stylists in most major cities who can provide you with in-home wardrobe consulting services. Contact us to get started today! service@DRESsystem.com

The Power of DRES Authors

Brenda Azevedo	Sacramento, CA	brenda@justbcosmetics.com
Colleen Bradley	Austin, TX	colleen@cbwardrobeconsulting.com
Kira Brown	Phoenix, AZ	kira@fashionphoenix.com
Lori Goddard-Weed	Everett, WA	imageisit@gmail.com
Cheryl Michaels	Issaquah, WA	agelessstylecoach@gmail.com
Melissa Sabatine	Washington, D.C.	melissa@capitolrunway.com
Kat Smith	Portland, OR	meaningfuljourney@gmail.com
Margaret Spencer	Seattle, WA	ms@dressystem.com
Corey Urbina	Greenville, SC	corey@stylemattersgreenville.com

DRES System Consulting

The DRES System offers personal style education for improved confidence and clarity. Let us help you curate your clothing collection to create the wardrobe of your dreams. At DRESsystem.com, we have put together the ultimate tools and support everyone needs to feel and look confident.

There are two options for involvement with the DRES System: online and in-person. For those of you who are more of the DIY type, we offer an online assessment of your DRES Profile, DRES Stylist online consulting, plus personal shopping that offers personalized recommendations. For the person who desires in-person service, we have a national network of talented DRES System–Certified Personal Stylists who are located in most major U.S. cities for in-home consulting appointments.

DRES Club Membership

Membership allows you to receive clothing recommendations for your body shape. You can work with our stylists online to stay up-to-date each season with outfit recommendations that are personally selected just for you by a DRES Stylist of your choosing. Each recommendation will be appropriate for your personal online profile. There is no commitment to purchase any recommended clothing items, though our recommendations come with links to easily find where to buy each item. Join now to get a free membership at DRESsystem.com.

DRES System–Certified Personal Stylists

From in-home consultations to personal shopping, there is nothing like the warmth of working with a friendly personal stylist who cares for you and will keep you looking your best.

In order to join our team of personal stylists and become certified in our DRES System, you must first take our comprehensive training program, complete fieldwork, and pass our exam. Many of our personal stylists have previous experience and bring with them extensive knowledge in a variety of areas.

Each stylist in our national network is an independent business owner. Schedule a free introductory call to find the personal stylist with the best fit or contact us for help in finding a DRES System–Certified Personal Stylist in your area at DRESsystem.com.

DRES SERVICES

Empowering Three-Step Consulting Process

Our process has essential steps to provide you with the best service possible. Profile, Organize, Shop is our three-step consulting process. With a smooth flow, one step to the next, the consulting process once completed equips you with the information, tools, and support you need to have a balanced wardrobe that brings out your brilliance.

Profile

It all starts with the profile. The only way to build the ultimate wardrobe is by starting with the right foundation. Here, we help to define your fashion style, color range, and your body's unique proportions. We assess your lifestyle and clothing needs. This service includes our DRES StyleGuide, which is a style book personalized just for you. A custom color palette can be added to this service for your ultimate forty-two colors.

"It's not the money that makes you well dressed, it's understanding."
—Christian Dior, fashion designer

Color Assessment

We'll bring out your brilliance by defining your forty-two Ultimate Colors out of over five hundred! We use our exclusive DRES System colors to provide a detailed assessment of your individual coloring and create a personalized Color Palette.

Organize

Nothing can be purchased before we know what you already have. We work with you to edit your wardrobe, narrowing it down to your best pieces. Through this process and the profile, we advise you on your missing pieces with a shopping list to round out your wardrobe. Your closet is now well organized and sorted into categories and looking like a personal boutique.

"True elegance consists not in having a closet bursting with clothes, but rather in having a few well-chosen numbers in which one feels totally at ease."
—Coco Chanel

Shop

Now that we have a shopping list, we can help you track down the best items that fit your profile. Personal shopping can be done for you and delivered to you, or we can guide you on a private shopping experience.

Outfit Styling

Your Stylist will show you how to coordinate and document outfits from your wardrobe. You'll receive a beautiful photo catalog to easily reference your best looks.

Face Styling

We'll determine your facial proportions and discuss the best way to dress your face to complement your features. Discover the best hairstyles, glasses, accessories, and makeup for your face shape and proportions.

"Women usually love what they buy,
yet hate two-thirds of what is in their closets."
—Mignon McLaughlin, journalist/author

Wardrobe Update

Refresh your wardrobe before each new season by clearing out the old and bringing in the new. Your stylist will work with you to incorporate new trends that are appropriate for you, help you get organized, and create new outfits for the season ahead.

Special Occasions

Need help finding the perfect outfit for a wedding, black-tie event, business meeting, or reunion? Maybe you need help packing for your whole trip. We can help you put together a complete outfit that is perfect so that you can look and feel your best.

Shopping Tours

Are you traveling to a new city on business or pleasure? If you have a few hours, contact one of our DRES System–Certified Stylists to put together a personalized tour. We'll save you time by taking you directly to the best boutiques in the city that are just your style.

DRES TOOLS

DRES Tools are exclusively available through the DRESsystem.com website and our DRES System–Certified Personal Stylists. They are included during private in-home consulting appointments and designed to bring clarity to your wardrobe selections.

StyleGuide

This personalized StyleGuide is a book that's customized for you by your DRES Stylist. It holds your unique shopping profile in a beautiful silver clutch purse. Included in the Profile appointment.

StyleGuide Inserts

With most of our additional services, StyleGuide Inserts are added to your StyleGuide for further personalization.

Color Palette Insert and Color Codes

Just like a custom-made painting, the personalized color palette holds fabric swatches of your forty-two Ultimate Colors and is included in the Color Assessment appointment. Another option is a pre-made Color Code fan.

StyleLog

Imagine browsing through a catalog of all of your best outfits, designed by your DRES Stylist and featuring you as the model! Included in the Outfit Styling appointment.

StyleTabs

When we leave you with an organized and edited wardrobe, your closet's look will make you feel like you're walking into an organized boutique. Included in our Organize appointment.

WHAT PEOPLE SAY

"The DRES System wardrobe makeover was a wonderful experience for me. At first I was a little nervous about inviting someone into my house to do an in-depth look at my body shape and my clothes. But once we began, the whole thing was easy and comfortable. The change in my confidence has been apparent to my family, friends, and co-workers, and I encourage every woman to have an honest, helpful guide who can show you how to look beautiful and dress well, no matter what your shape or size. Thank you DRES System."
—Erica Gaddis, Client SD3 (Sapphire, Dramatic, Color Code 3)

Empowering women with more self-confidence is the main reason the DRES System exists. It's fun and rewarding. Once you see the power in showing a woman her beauty, you want to do it again. It's rewarding to know that she will spread that joy to her family and community.

"Although I had a closet full of clothes, I still always found myself standing there overwhelmed and frustrated that I could never find anything to wear! The DRES System helped me better understand what styles and colors best compliment me. I realize now that I do not have to hide behind "maternity-style" shirts anymore; I feel more confident wearing clothes that best accentuate my body shape. The DRES System is a very useful guide and has helped make shopping for clothes a more enjoyable experience."
—Julie Raupp, Client RE12 (Ruby, Ethnic, Color Color 12)

Sometimes we get tears of joy once we complete the last step of the Profile, Organize, Shop process. Typically, our clients have never seen themselves in this light where they feel so beautiful. We later get letters of gratitude where they share with us all the compliments they get from friends and coworkers. It's not only what is transforming on the outside, it's also what is transforming on the inside that enhances beauty.

"They helped me 'think outside the box' and guided me toward pieces I may not have ever chosen on my own. Their experienced eyes saved me a lot of time. I'm so glad I did this! I know I learned how to make better choices and spend my money wisely for future purchases."

—Karen Herrema, Student EC11 (Emerald, Chic, Color Code 11)

Even our students who go through our DRES Stylist certification course are unexpectedly transformed and look more brilliant. This goes to show that even a fashion-conscious person can benefit from the DRES System. My belief is that everyone would gain power from knowing their DRES Code and having a DRES Personal Stylist!

Join the DRES Club at **www.DRESsystem.com**

ACKNOWLEDGMENTS

A huge thank you to Nancy Hogan for being my partner on this book project, I could not have done it without you! Your witty sense of humor always kept me laughing through late evenings of editing while we were still in our pajamas.

A big shout-out to our fabulous proofreader, Carrie Wicks, for her masterful attention to detail.

I also want to recognize all the talented personal stylists I've had the opportunity to work with. I appreciate the dedication and creativity you bring to this industry and your passion for helping women feel confident. It has been a great joy for me to watch your businesses grow and develop over the years.

To all the clients who have used the DRES System, thank you for your willingness to learn and for supporting the empowerment of women.

My supportive husband Andy and my younger daughter Emma also deserve a big thanks for giving me the time to work the extra hours needed to complete this book project.

Lastly, I'd like to thank my brilliant daughter Cleo for helping me during her last summer at home before heading off to college. From your editing and formatting assistance to your advice and moral support, you have helped me make this book a success.

With warmest regards,
Margaret Spencer

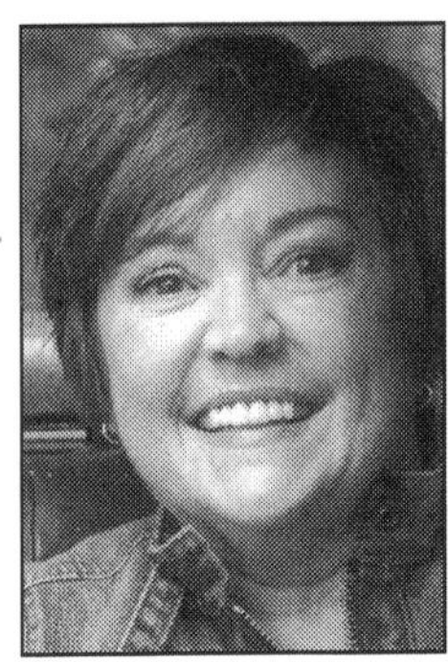

Nancy Hogan

Primary Editor and Book Project Manager

NancyEdits, l.l.c.
www.nancyedits.net
nancy@nancyedits.net
Edmonds, Washington

Nancy's obsession with words started early—precociously early.

She had wanted to major in liberal arts, but took her dad's advice to choose a career path offering independence. She was able to capitalize on those high school secretarial courses and paid her way through college.

Ready to get out into the world, she started her work life as secretary to the program director of KABC TalkRadio in Los Angeles. Her career in show business saw her through eight fun years and gave her the chance to meet and work with some creative, fascinating people. For her last gig in L.A., Nancy worked for Mel Brooks as his script secretary on *The History of the World—Part I.* If you ask her, she might even tell you which joke is hers.

Nancy followed her love for words, editing, and writing into publications, marketing, and advertising. Ready for change, she moved to Seattle in 1987, where her favorite job was licensing photography as a virtual sales consultant with Getty Images, achieving over one million dollars in sales in both 2002 and 2003, during a huge advertising downturn.

Seattle has been good to Nancy. After marrying the Best Husband in the World, she refreshed her editing skills via the University of Washington Editing Certificate Program; and now serves on their advisory board.

She launched NancyEdits in 2009, and loves to make your words bright and snappy.